26 95

D0850207

VISION IN
THE ANIMAL WORLD

VISION IN
THE ANIMAL WORLD

R. H. Smythe, M.R.C.V.S.

First published 1975 by

THE MACMILLAN PRESS LTD.
London and Basingstoke
Associated companies in New York Dublin Melbourne
Johannesburg and Madras

SBN 333 18034 8

Printed by Thomson Litho Ltd, East Kilbride, Scotland

CONTENTS

Introduction   viii
Chapter 1 : What is vision?   1
    Light and vision   3
    Visual needs in the animal kingdom and how   6
      they developed
    The art of seeing   9
Chapter 2 : The mammalian eye   15
    Distance perception in other animals compared 21
      with mammals
    Parallax and parallactic displacement   22
    Eye movements   23
    Colour vision   27
    Day and night vision   28
    Night blindness   30
Chapter 3 : The human eye   31
    The lid-closure reflex   32
    The conjunctiva   33
    Accommodation   38
    The cornea   38
    Aqueous humour   42
    The sclerotic coat or sclera   44
    The choroid coat   46
    Movements of the eyeball   46
    The optic lens   46
    The iris   47
    Intraocular pressure in man and other animals 48
    The retina   50
    Construction of the retina   55
    Rods and cones   57

Chapter 4: The eye of the dog   60
            The palpebral fissure   60
            The cornea   61
            The lens   62
            The retina   62
            The iris   64
            Accommodation in mammals   65
            Vision in the dog   72
Chapter 5: The eye of the cat   75
Chapter 6: The eye of the horse   80
            The eyeball   81
            Vision in the horse   84
            The iris   84
            The crystalline lens   85
            The eyelids   85
            The tapetum   86
            The membrananictitans   86
            Accommodation   87
Chapter 7: Vision in other mammals   91
            Other ungulates   91
            The elephant   93
            The rhinoceros   93
            The hippopotamus   93
            The whale   94
            The seal   95
Chapter 8: Vision in birds   96
            The eyes of birds   96
Chapter 9: The eyes of fishes   107
Chapter 10: Vision in reptiles and some aquatic animals   114
            Lizards   115
            Slow worms   116
            Chameleons   116
            Crocodiles and alligators   116
            Tortoises, terrapins and turtles   117
            Aquatic creatures: frogs, toads and newts   117
Chapter 11: Vision in insects and spiders   119
            Compound eyes   121
            Colour perception through compound eyes   123
            Dorsal ocelli   123
            The cornea of an ocellus   124

Function 124
Lateral ocelli 126
Spiders 127
Chapter 12: Miscellaneous animals—notes on special 129
   peculiarities
    Amoeba 129
    Anteater 129
    Apes 129
    Bats 130
    Beavers 130
    Bittern 130
    Bleak 130
    Dogfish 130
    Flying foxes and fruit bats 130
    The guacharo bird 132
    Gurnard 132
    Herring 132
    Kiwi 132
    Mole 132
    Opossum 132
    Otter 133
    Rodents 133
    The spectral tarsier 134
    Trout 134
    Vultures 134
    Water voles and rats 134
    Worms 135
    Crabs, lobsters, shrimps and prawns 135
    Snails and slugs 137
    Octopuses and squids 137
    Oysters and limpets 137
Chapter 13: What do animals see? 140
    Parallax 157
    Movement in insects 157
Bibliography 160
Index 161

INTRODUCTION

The world is full of eyes. We are unaware of the presence or the existence of most of them although they may be all around us. The probability is that the majority of these eyes do not see us either, or at least not sufficiently well to enable their owners to determine whether or not we are living objects unless, of course, we move.

Any change in the relative position of one body to another is sufficient to attract attention and give rise to action.

Although such activity is frequently reflex in its nature, it is none the less a defence mechanism, and one which has helped to maintain world population. Creatures which lack social protection, learn to move first and think later. They live longer that way. Humanity is apt to regard the world as a place designed especially for its own delectation. It worships a Maker whom it fondly imagines to be a larger or more erudite replica of itself. Throughout the world there exist hundreds of millions of other creatures, huge or microscopic, which for all we know, may quite justly entertain the same idea. Many of the more lowly among these see no creatures other than their own kind. Others, more highly developed, see a variety of the world's inhabitants, with varying degrees of clarity and definition. But, on the whole, practically all living animals with any degree of discrimination, regard the world as a place bathed in sunshine in which they can move around, mix with their fellows and discover through their eyes, all the food and drink and comforts which make existence worthwhile. Whether or not they may be harbouring a delusion, is quite another matter.

The eye is an optical instrument and it may be presumed that there would be no such thing as radio or television had the eye never come into being, and unless, of course, we were able to acquire the machinery capable of translating light rays into what we now recognise as vision, and other rays into sound. Nor would we be capable of recognising light had we not been born with a specially built-in apparatus, able to convert wavelengths into energy, together with an optical instrument known as the eye, which is able to translate such impressions into vision with the co-operation furnished by a specially developed portion of the brain.

Herein lies one of the great mysteries associated with life: had not vision been granted to its inmates, the world would be empty of all but the most primitive creatures. One question which arises is: Did animals come into being with a fully-tested, working visual outfit, primitive as it may have been? Or, did those in which the elements of vision originally existed, gradually, by a process of survival of the fittest, slowly improve their built-in apparatus until it achieved its present state of near perfection?

A brain, however highly developed, would have been quite useless unless it contained this specially developed area which enables visual impressions conveyed to the retina by light waves (short electro-magnetic waves) to be translated into the visual image. The two elements: stimulation by energy from the light waves and the apparatus for interpretation, had to exist in the same organism in the same degree of perfection, in order that life might be maintained on earth.

As well as the animal kingdom, vegetation of nearly every variety depends for its existence upon those same wavelengths which enable us to see the rate of its growth, and note changes in the colouration of its foliage. Possibly the sunbather who lies with the body exposed upon the beach in summer, with eyes shielded by dark glasses, can provide evidence of the effect of light rays direct from the sun, upon the human body. The limpet on the rock, and the worm upon the lawn, possess no evident brains, but they carry light spots or dermal receptors on portions of their body surfaces—small areas sensitive to light rays—and when these become stimulated, both creatures become aware that such portions of their bodies are exposed and have become vulnerable to enemy attack.

When one studies the eyes of different animals and tries to estimate exactly how much each is able to see: whether it has the power to focus objects clearly and whether it sees the world in black and white, or in colour, one cannot avoid being amazed at the great differences which exist in eyes throughout the animal kingdom.

It becomes apparent that each individual species has different requirements and that the visual apparatus of each is specially adapted to its needs and its limitations. This is what one might really expect since the ability of any animal to survive depends upon the sensual organs with which it is equipped, as well as upon its ability to react appropriately when the need arises. The survivors probably had acquired some slight improvement over their ancestors in the matter of sight and hearing, just as much as in athletic ability, and so the improvements became genetically established.

The interesting point is the very many different directions in which progress has been made. The eyes of a bird would be as useless to a rat as those of the rat to the bird. Then again, the visual apparatus has to be specially adapted to the environment in which the animal lives: some animals live in the air more than upon the ground; some prefer bright light while others tend to live more or less in darkness, some live on land and in water while others live on the water or underneath its surface. Each requires an entirely different, but specialised, type of eye and visual characteristics. The miracle, if it may be so styled, is that each animal has in the way of eye structure, exactly what it needs.

In the following chapters we will endeavour to determine the various kinds of eyes, how they function and how well they are adapted to the needs of their owners.

CHAPTER 1

WHAT IS VISION?

In days gone by the eye was regarded as 'the gateway to the brain'!

As soon as life developed throughout the world and animals were compelled to move from place to place, eyes became an essential part of their anatomy. They were necessary not only for the purpose of finding food but also to provide warning of attack. In our own lives the possession of vision gives us essential information concerning the relationship between our bodies and surrounding objects. It enables us to pass between them, or over them, or around them, as the case may be.

We can determine by using our eyes, whether the objects we perceive are close to us or far away, and whether they are stationary or moving. Movement is detectable when the distance between any two objects varies continuously, or intermittently. Gradually, as the result of experience, we learn the types of object which may prove dangerous and how soon to move away from their vicinity. We decide, by our sense of touch, whether the objects are solid, hard or soft, dry or wet after we have verified their presence and made up our minds whether it is safe to approach them.

Human beings not only observe objects in the mass but they possess an ability to endow them with colour. All animals are not so lucky: the dog, for example, sees all objects in shades of grey, in much the same way that we see similar shades and tones in a black-and-white photographic print. Many people who keep dogs will dispute this statement and maintain that their own dog knows at once whether its mistress is wearing her bright red dress which it much prefers, or her mauve one, which for some reason it does not appreciate. A pet monkey could distinguish between these two frocks, the one from the other, instantly, because it possesses full colour vision, as we do. The dog, however, sees them only in tones of greyness but it can

1

differentiate them since the one frock is a very dark grey and the other ever so much lighter in tone.

We ourselves can derive a great deal of information from studying a black-and-white print, partly because we know from experience the natural colouring, and in our minds, if need be, we can translate the greyness into its natural colours; although in most instances we are quite content to observe its form only.

Our own eyes are essential to our well-being, if only to enable us to go from place to place in safety—or nowadays in comparative safety—and in order that we may carry out the activities essential to the maintenance of existence. But to a recently born infant, or to a puppy a fortnight old, with its eyes only recently opened, objects focussed onto the retina—the light sensitive membrane at the back of the eyeball, which receives the visual image—convey a limited message.

The child, if its eyes are normal, will be able to recognise its mother by vision quite soon, but the puppy will know the whereabouts of its mother initially purely through its sense of smell. Other objects, including its litter companions, will mean practically nothing to it visually until after the fourth or fifth week of its life. It will need to come into actual contact with objects in the world other than itself. It will then be a matter of weeks before it begins to understand whether such objects are solid or soft, light or heavy, moving or stationary, living or inanimate.

The child may be six to nine weeks old before it recognises its mother's face in any visual detail, and this is demonstrated when Baby commences to smile. Nevertheless, at this time of its life it exhibits equal pleasure if any rounded object is held over its cot, as it does when its mother bends over it. The power of accommodation is not yet developed. The first thing it really recognises at a distance, is its bottle; and the first thing the puppy recognises and snuggles up to, is its food bowl.

But even in the latter case it is not just vision that enables the puppy to locate the bowl. The ability arises from its remarkable sense of smell, something no baby will ever possess in anything like the same degree. In a great many of the animals, which in a state of nature catch and kill their own food, this sense of smell appears to be as valuable as vision, and in some cases even more so. This, no doubt, is why so many aged dogs are kept as pensioners long after their sight has disappeared, since they still find their way about the house and garden; while some will continue to hunt in the fields and woods nearly as successfully as in the days when they could see. A blind man, without a dog to guide him, would be compelled to depend upon touch and hearing.

The domestic cat has an excellent sense of vision but has not the dog's remarkable faculty of smell. It is one of the quadrupeds which uses its two fore feet as though they were hands. A kitten in the nest, after its eyes have opened, endeavouring to learn a little more about the outside world, will touch a strange object very gently with the palm and digits of one fore foot. After this, it will grasp it between the palms of both fore feet and finally try biting it gently to discover whether it is hard or soft, and especially if it be good to eat. Having completed its investigation along these lines it will be in a better position to depend upon vision if it again encounters a similar object. In cats, as in humans, visual recognition is seldom immediately automatic so far as interpretation and understanding are concerned. The eyes have to be educated. Interpretation of the visual image is something which has to be learned, like a language. Cats catch mice almost entirely by a combination of vision and acrobatics, but dogs catch rats and rabbits chiefly by using the nose. There are, however, two types of hunting dog: those which favour vision and those which depend almost entirely upon scent. The Greyhound (a prominent member of the large family of 'gaze hounds'), hunts almost entirely by sight. Nevertheless, I have on more than one occasion observed an old, completely blind greyhound, alone in the fields after dark, hunting a hare and following its trail entirely with its nose.

This is strong evidence that the Greyhound possesses the ability to hunt either by sight (when its vision is good) or by scent, but that it prefers sight. On the other hand, the Foxhound and Beagle, the Bloodhound and the Spaniels, rely entirely upon smell; even when the quarry would be quite visible if the nose were lifted from the ground.

LIGHT AND VISION

Put briefly, vision provides the ability to recognise rays of light reaching the earth by radiation from the sun, as well as the capability of appreciating the effects such rays produce when they encounter earthly objects. Without eyes, the existence of light rays would not be apparent. Light and darkness exist only in the eyes of the beholder. Radiation implies the transfer of energy to the Earth by means of electro-magnetic waves. The sun radiates energy in the form of short, visible, rays of light, and longer, invisible rays of heat.

When light rays make contact with a solid object, they may behave in several ways: they may become almost entirely absorbed by the object, according to its structure; or they may be partly absorbed and partly reflected. It is through the reflected portion that our eyes receive a complete picture of the object; its dimension, texture and colour.

Refraction results when light passes through a transparent object and its rays are thus scattered and altered in direction.

Reflection occurs when light rays are only partly absorbed and the remainder are deflected away from the surface to form the basis of the perception of an object. Extreme intensity of illumination can cause dazzle and poor perception of the object by the viewer, but in most instances the reflection from anything but a bright or polished surface is mild and our eyes are able to form a definite impression of it. This impression is transmitted along the nerves travelling to the part.of the brain which translates it into a visual image.

When the object upon which the rays fall possesses several surfaces set on different planes, each able to absorb, reflect or scatter the rays, certain surface planes will reflect some of the light waves back and into our eyes, eventually providing us with a visual image. But a few surfaces may be so situated that they do not receive the rays, which are in some way blocked off. These areas will remain unilluminated, giving rise to what we describe as a 'shadow'.

The contrast between lighted areas and those in shadow will produce in trained eyes a definite image which the brain can interpret into what we all recognise as conformation, or to put it more simply — 'shape'.

It is this ability of the brain to carry out such interpretation which enables vision to attain its final stage of perfection.

It will be gathered that light and darkness are not real and separate states, apart from the fact that they become translated by a combination of the eyes and the brain into distinct visual images. In other words, both light and darkness are the products of our visual perception.

In reality light is simply an abstract quality existent only in the mind of man or any other animal capable of appreciating it. There is no such thing as light apart from a mental impression conveyed to the brain through the medium of the eyes. As G. L. Walls wrote (*The Vertebrate Eye*, 1942) 'We have been discussing light as an objective, physical entity. Just as there would be no sound if a tree were to fall with nobody to hear it, so also there would be no light in the physiological sense if there were no photo-receptor upon which it impinged. In this sense light is a sensation, an experience in consciousness.'

The visual spectrum embraces wavelengths between 4000 Å and 7600 Å. (1 Angström $= 10^{-8}$ cm.) Waves shorter than 4000 Å are known as ultraviolet rays and those over 7600 Å are infra-red. Nevertheless, the retina of man is sensitive to wavelengths well out-side these limits. Walls showed that in man, insensitivity of the eye to ultraviolet light up to 3500 Å, is entirely due to absorption by the lens of the eye. Aphakic subjects (those who have had the lens surgically removed), are able to see quite easily through these wave-lengths, calling the sensation either blue or violet. In other instances, the retina may be abnormally sensitive to red light and such individuals may be able to evoke visual sensitivity to wavelengths greater than 7600 Å. Some of the birds of prey, notably hawks and owls are capable of detecting infra-red rays emanating from the bodies of mice, rabbits and birds by night, when it would be impossible to recognise their whereabouts by means of the usually accepted wavelengths.

To make this a little easier to understand, let us now consider what happens in the case of radio or television. When speech, a piece of music, or a television picture are broadcast from a station, each enters space in the form of electro-magnetic waves, similar to light waves, but differing in their respective wavelengths. A person sitting in a room a hundred miles away from a broadcasting station can in no way sense or feel the presence of these waves until a suitable receiving apparatus converts them into what we recognise as music, speech or a picture.

We would not be conscious of light rays (apart from the possible presence of accompanying heat waves) unless we were provided with a suitable receiving apparatus, which in this case is the eye acting in co-operation with the brain, which translates the stimuli conveyed by the light waves into a visual image.

VISUAL NEEDS IN THE ANIMAL KINGDOM AND HOW THEY DEVELOPED

In the world of today the answer would seem obvious. It has now become a centre of hurry and it appears to be essential for most people to be able to travel from one place to another as quickly as possible. To do this safely, one must be able to see very well indeed. But as far as man is concerned, his unaided eyes are no better and no worse than they were two thousand years ago, in spite of the fact that his environment and his optical needs have changed entirely. The one thing in its favour is that the human eye happens to be one of the simplest of all eyes and it has very little that may go wrong with it which cannot now be corrected by surgery, or by providing artificial appendages, much in the same way that one acquires artificial teeth.

Sight became especially important to man when he developed the upright position during his evolutionary development. Prior to this, he bore the lengthy arms of the primates, but when he commenced to stand upright on two legs, his arms became shorter. This was of considerable assistance in that it facilitated holding and manipulating objects between his flexible fingers, to bring them within range of his eyes so that he might see them clearly by his binocular vision. Subsequently, he began to invent tools, but the danger point in man's history was when he first became aware of a round tree trunk rolling down a hill. From this, the wheel was born. Considering all the things to which man has become accustomed, one might regard the wheel as an unmitigated blessing to his kind. But one must remember that the wheel has made it possible for him to move at speeds far higher than those with which his vision can cope and at the same time maintain a state of safety.

The conflict between rapidity of movement and clarity of vision has cost more in human lives throughout the past fifty years than all the wars in history.

A dog, a cat and a hippopotamus, can go throughout life without their eyesight being questioned, even if it deteriorates somewhat through age, sickness, or accident. In man, frequent visits to the oculist and optician provide him with artificial aids which overcome difficulties as they arise. But man is dependent almost solely upon his vision, while most other animals make considerable use of some of their other senses, particularly the sense of smell; while a number

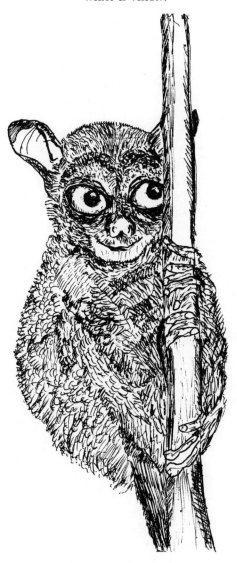

Fig. 1   The Tarsier. The Primate with the largest eyes in relation
to body size among all animals.

get along quite well with very poor vision, or even with no eyes at all. Naturally their noses are nearer the ground than ours, in a great many instances. If the need for vision exists in a tall animal, such as a giraffe, the neck is usually sufficiently long to bring the eyes close to earth. None of the earliest forms of primitive life were provided with vision, which developed through the ages as a consequence of general evolution.

During this evolution, the first eyes possessing characteristics comparable with modern eyes probably appeared in the amphibious age, when animals made use of them on land and under water. Later they became adapted to use on dry ground, when our ancestors found it was easier to crawl out of the water and enjoy the more plentiful produce of the land. All this happened about five hundred million years ago.

Those familiar with the oft quoted remark, 'Do you think I have eyes in the back of my head?' may be surprised to hear that their ancestors actually possessed something of this nature. There is one little swimming creature which still carries a solitary eye. It is known as *Cyclops*. Infants of various species are sometimes born with a single eye and in one instance a horse possessing one enormous central eye, grew to maturity. This is a rare congenital condition, not dependent upon evolutionary reversion.

Sometimes the two eyes are fused into one; in other cases a central median eye may lie between two normal eyes. Some of the invertebrates—the king crabs—possess a strange organ known as a 'median eye', placed centrally between the eyes proper. On top of the brain of every fish, frequently anchored by a long stalk, is the vestigial remains of a third eye, known as the pineal body. It is possible that during the earlier stages of evolution, fishes carried a row of eyes on top of each head. As the laterally placed eyes developed, these dorsal eyes became smaller and eventually they disappeared. Two pairs of these pineal eyes remained in the lampreys until fairly recent times—probably only a few million years ago.

The pineal body appears to have been of considerable importance as an actual sense organ in the earliest vertebrates, mainly because an animal feeding under water, say on the bottom of a lake, would be able to ascertain what was going on at a higher level; possibly on the surface of the water. It therefore assisted in the survival and maintenance of the vertebrates. In the lampreys of today, rays of light still reach this third eye through a slit in the surface of the skull and focus onto an elementary retina. It is hardly likely that the lampreys are able to see with this eye but nevertheless the eye remains sensitive to light. The lamprey is one of those creatures susceptible to colour changes in the skin of the body, creating a type of camouflage, and it is possible that this third eye, or what remains of it enables this creature to vary its body colour in accordance with its environment at any particular time. The Tuatera lizard of New Zealand, a rather sluggish nocturnal creature, often referred to as the Sphenodon, has a functional medial eye, capable of some degree of visual discrimination. This has resulted from fusion of the two original eyes.

Many of the extinct amphibians also possessed medial eyes but these have long since disappeared, though the frog is said 'to carry a jewel in its head'. Probably this legend relates to a small cystic structure beneath the skin of the forehead which is still easy to find. This is probably all that remains of it's third eye. Birds do not appear to have retained this third eye, or at least they show no vestige of it. In birds and mammals generally, including ourselves, the only vestige remaining is the pineal body, which lies in the posterior wall of the third ventricle of the brain, immediately above the pons and between this and the upper portion of the cerebellum.

THE ART OF SEEING

Quite frequently we stare at an object some little distance from us and our brain presents a picture for consideration. We may repeat the observation on several occasions and find that our recording shows some slight variation.

Most of us see when we wish to do so, but our recording is sometimes tempered by what we wish to see. In an art gallery you may be accompanied by a friend and may both view the same picture. To you this may appear to represent a Cyclops with one eye, several ears, half a nose and a variety of scattered limbs. You would describe the effect if you were asked, in colloquial terms, as 'a bit of a mess'. Your friend, quite enthralled by the composition and its implications, will assure you that it is a brilliant impression of a famous ballet dancer, and you hear later that the picture has changed hands for what you would regard as a small fortune. What one sees is purely a matter of one's own interpretation.

As I remarked earlier, a lot of animals get along quite well without eyes, or at least without vision. Horses and cattle, rats, mice, rabbits, stoats, weasels, hedgehogs and fish, to mention only a few, may get by even when completely blind, escape possible enemies and find sufficient food to avoid starvation over long periods. Moles have primitive eyes and little or no vision but their lives are spent mainly underground searching for worms which have no eyes at all. Vision, in areas where no light waves can penetrate, would be impracticable.

It is well known that the inhabitants of the waters of deep underground caves and lakes are almost invariably blind, and as they arrived in such situations after these had lost any possibility of illumination, it can only be surmised that any fish or other creature that became trapped within their depths arrived with two functional eyes but that their ultimate descendants developed blindness mainly because there was no use for vision, and an inherited blindness was no longer a reason for extermination as it would have been in a world of light.

It has been shown by recent experiments, mainly with crippled animals, that the inheritance of a fault such as blindness, is only 25 per cent the result of heredity, and 75 per cent the issue of environment, and attendant consequences.

Dogs which become blind following a period during which they enjoy normal vision, find their way about their house and garden entirely by smell. On a farm, a blind dog will trace its way out and back home by following its own scent. Some small, blind, pet dogs will even gallop after and retrieve a ball thrown across the lawn. But most blind dogs become a little lost if the furniture in the house is frequently changed in position.

But, although the human eye has remained practically unchanged through the ages, man's brain has changed in a remarkable fashion. It has enabled him to make use of the information he receives from his vision and to turn it to extraordinary uses—good, bad and questionable.

G. L. Walls, in his *Vertebrate Eye*, points out that human vision, so valuable and so kaleidoscopic, is the product of a complex brain teamed with a remarkably simple eye. We must not assume that more complex eyes (always connected with simpler brains), afford their owners anything so informative of the environment as does the vision we experience.

Eyes which became too efficient might raise problems and cause their owner a deal of embarrassment. Man has overcome this possibility by seeing a lot but observing only a very little. If he walks the length of a street, engaged with his own thoughts, he will probably see several hundred people. If he were asked at the end of the street to describe any of the people he had encountered and actually noticed, it is more than likely that he would be quite unable to recall any one of them or describe whom or what he had seen in anything but very general terms. But it might happen that one person he met was of considerable interest and the impression he had registered of that person might enable him to describe him, or her, in great detail. His eye is merely an optical instrument. It is not the eye that sees but the brain behind it. The eye merely observes and the brain behind it decides whether or not to develop the picture.

Whether visual acuity is of particular importance to any variety of animal depends mainly upon two factors:

(a) The kind of environment in which the animal is compelled, or chooses to live. This may be above or under water, in bright light or in darkness.

(b) The way by which an animal manages to maintain its existence. This concerns the way in which it contrives to catch, or in some other way obtain the kind of food it requires. Birds and bats, the one operating mainly in daylight and the other in comparative darkness, both of them compelled at times to catch and consume their food in mid-air, require exceptionally acute vision of a specialised type. Other varieties of birds may depend equally upon acuity of vision to enable them to see at long range objects upon the ground which may possess a food value. A buzzard, for example, soaring some two or three hundred feet above open country, will be quite capable of recognising a mouse crouching upon the ground, or even moving among short undergrowth, and will be able to retain the moving mouse within its vision while it dives to earth to make the kill.

An owl might do nearly as well by night but would be far less capable in bright sunlight, although some species of owls do sometimes hunt in daylight. Other animals which hunt both by day and by night, such as the cats, are almost equally capable in bright light or in near darkness. We will read about all these matters later, especially when we learn about the iris and the pupil of the eye, and its ability, in some animals at least, to adapt itself so as to lessen the amount of light entering the eye, or to increase this to the full

during the hours of comparative darkness. Some of the animals that
fly by night ot live in caves devoid of light, have a special apparatus
working on the principle of radar. By producing sound vibrations
they are able to register the recoil of these from solid objects, into
which they might otherwise fly. The echo from prominences, walls
and ceilings, keeps bats informed as to the distance between them
and such obstacles, in time for them to avoid them.

Many other creatures depend upon feelers, which may take the
form of antennae, or even whiskers. Insects are generally provided
with sensitive antennae, not only in front but even all over the body
surface. The domestic cat would be completely at a loss if some
misguided individual trimmed off its whiskers. It is said that the cat
can pass through a space or a hole in a fence or hedge which is not
less in diameter than that of its crop of whiskers. Without them,
its ability to calculate such distance would be seriously impaired.

In the case of the arthropods and crustaceans as represented by
the shrimps and prawns, the lobsters and the crabs, as well as in the
snails, we find stalked eyes. Apart from the snails, many of these
creatures are provided with antennae also. Even some flies carry eyes
on stalks.

Some of the feelers, especially among insects, and mosquitoes in
particular, are capable of sending out signals and receiving messages
in Morse fashion. It is recorded that a male mosquito is able to make
contact with a female a mile distant purely as the result of vibratory
messages sent and received. The ability of the male to see his
prospective mate only comes into force when he is within two feet of
her. These antennae have an additional function which makes vision
a matter of minor importance. The mosquito female needs a feed of
blood before she can establish her fertility. To secure this she flies
around until her antennae register the warmth issuing from a human
body some feet away. She has no need to recognise the body visually,
her antennae provide all the information she requires.

Not only mosquitoes, but animals in general, do not use vision to
distinguish between the sexes. When two dogs meet in midwinter
when the oestrous cycle is generally dormant in the female, neither
recognises the sex of the other in spite of structural differences which
would be obvious to the human eye. Instead, the two will gallop
past one another and while so doing each will take a quick sniff at
the other's body. This is invariably sufficient to decide whether their
future relationship will result in courtship or battle.

Birds and a good many other animals make a study of behaviour to determine sex, and in such cases vision has its obvious uses. Courtship display, as well as colour, is taken notice of by birds, snakes, dolphins and certain fishes, to mention only a few of the animals that employ vision as an aid to sex determination.

It has recently been shown that light received through the eyes has a definite influence upon fertility. Female quadrupeds kept in darkness are slow to exhibit oestrus, or may fail to do so at all. When it does make its appearance the desire to mate is diminished, and when mating takes place the chances of conception are lessened. Alternatively, when sheep are exported to countries where the seasons are opposed to our own, a general upset in the breeding cycle may occur. When they leave here early in winter and arrive in a land of sunshine they come into oestrus and breed when they would have remained sexually dormant in their own country. Similarly, going from an English summer to a land where it is winter, with short days, may delay oestrus, so that the animals exhibit no sign of it and a delay in their breeding cycle results.

Fishes and those mammals which spend a great deal of their lives hunting their food beneath water level need a special type of eye and, at least in fishes, a differently shaped lens and a different method of focussing objects immersed in water. The goldfish, swimming in a circular bowl, can see objects in the water but it is unlikely it can see objects outside the glass of the bowl with any degree of definition. Under water in shallow lakes or pools, the occurence of reflection has an importance and the fish may actually see what is going on around or below it by looking at the reflection apparent on the underneath side of the water surface. We shall discuss this more later.

It is evident that in the animal world there exists not only a marked difference in visual responses but also an equally important difference in the structure of the eyes and in the nature of the work such eyes may be called upon to perform in a variety of circumstances. If we wonder why such a variety of eyes came into being, we must realise—as did Darwin—that only those creatures which possessed, or developed in the process of evolution, what one might almost regard as abnormalities (mutations), became able to survive and reproduce their kind. Those which retained or developed eyes of inferior quality soon became the victims of other animals and failed to reproduce, with the result that the inferior eyes disappeared and a more useful variety took their place.

The fact that a species remains in existence today after having held its place in the world for thousands or millions of years, proves that throughout its evolutionary career it has undergone salutary changes and used them to the best advantage.

CHAPTER 2

THE MAMMALIAN EYE

In the majority of carnivorous and herbivorous animals the eye is almost spherical, as in dog, cat and man.

The following dimensions may be of interest:

| | AXIS | | |
Animal	From front to back (mm)	Vertical (mm)	Transverse (mm)
Man	24·60	23·50	23·90
Dog (Fox Terrier)	19	20	20
Horse	44	50·50	54
Cat	21	21	21
Indian Elephant	30	33	35
Cow	37	42	43
Pig	22	24	25

In the vertebrates the eyeball is contained in, and surrounded to a large extent, by bone. The bony chamber which contains the eyeball is termed the *orbit*. The exposed portion of the eyeball comprises the cornea and some part of the sclerotic, while in many of the mammals, other than the Primates, the exposed portion can be protected, when protection is needed, by operating the third eyelid. Thomson Henderson in *Principles of Opthalmology* (1950), gives the following measurements of the cornea and eyeball in millimetres, selected from those of a large number of animals:

15

Animal	Transverse (mm)	Vertical (mm)	A-posterior (mm)
Horse			
Cornea	35	28·5	
Globe	54	50·5	44
Ox			
Cornea	29	24	
Globe	43	42	37
Pig			
Cornea	15·5	12·5	
Globe	25	24	22
Sheep			
Cornea	25	18·5	
Globe	34	33	31
Cat			
Cornea	16	15·5	21
Globe	21	21	21
Indian Elephant			
Cornea	23	20	
Globe	35	33	30
Camel			
Cornea	34	24	
Globe	47	45	40
Fox			
Cornea	15	15	
Globe	18	17	18
Black and Tan Terrier			
Cornea	13·5	13	
Globe	19·5	19·5	18·5
Retriever			
Cornea	17	16	
Globe	25	25	25

The depth and shape of the orbit differs in the various species and the amount of cover provided by the bony orbit, and particularly by its outer aspect. The orbital ring, is greater in some animals than in others. In domesticated animals the orbital ring varies in its completeness, according to the species, and accordingly the orbit is described as closed or open depending on whether the eyeball is entirely surrounded by an optic ring or only partially so.

The following is a list of animals and the type of orbit, open or closed, they possess:

Open	Closed
Bears	Primates including Man
Wolves	Horse family
Dogs	Domestic cattle
Foxes	Most of the Deer
Cats	Buffalo
Mink	Camel
Weasels	Moose
Otters	Musk Ox
Seals	Modern Teleost fishes
Rabbits and Hares	Turtles
Most rodents	Alligators and Crocodiles
Elephants	
Warthogs	
Marsupials	
Edentates	
Some of the Pigs	
Birds (except the Australian Cockatoo)	
Bats (usually)	
Frogs and Toads	
Snakes(except Boas and Pythons)	
Lizards (except Sphenodon)	
Sharks	

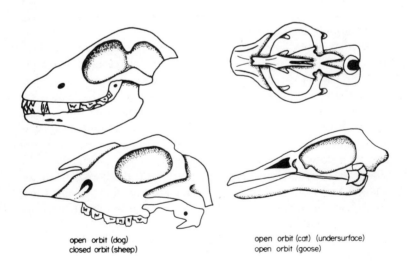

open orbit (dog)
closed orbit (sheep)

open orbit (cat) (undersurface)
open orbit (goose)

Fig. 2   The open and the closed orbit.

Most of the carniverous animals, including the dog family, although they lack a complete orbital ring, are provided with a considerable degree of eye protection by the presence of a well-developed zygomatic arch derived mainly from the malar bone. This bony arch projects and widens the face, thus reducing the risk of blows upon the eye. In the closed orbits the zygoma joins up with the frontal bone above to complete the orbit which contains only the eye. In the open orbit the cavity is not completely divided and it contains the eyeball in its anterior portion and the upper end of the ramus of the lower jaw in its posterior portion. (See Figure 2.)

Most of the animals, such as the dog, which possess the open orbit have the eye itself enclosed in a powerful orbital sheath. A ligament stretches across the orbit behind eye level and the eye is firmly attached to this. Nevertheless, in the brachycephalic or short-faced breed of dogs, such as the Pekinese, undue pressure or traction on the skin of the head or neck, may cause prolapse of the eyeball which may be forced out to lie on the cheek. In the cat the ligament is shorter and the orbital cavity is less distinctly divided into two parts, so in this animal prolapse of the eyeball is rare.

Before we discuss the eyes of other individual animals in detail it might be wise to look at the visual arrangements common to many of them. For example, let us first give attention to the third eyelid, or membrana nictitans. This has disappeared from the human eye, which may perhaps be unfortunate, as under the conditions in which men have to work in many trades it might still possess advantages. It is present in the horse and dog, in the ruminants, and in the birds. In the mammals thus endowed, the orbit contains a pad of fat underlying the eyeball. In the dog, for example, the third eyelid covers three-quarters of the eyeball when it is fully protruded. The only carnivorous mammal without it, is the skunk. In the horse and dog its presence can easily be demonstrated if one partly closes the lower lid and exerts pressure through it upon the eyeball with the tip of a finger. In the ox, it is larger and forms folds when caused to protrude in this way. Reindeer and Polar bears use it, together with the diving birds, as a complete, transparent window in place of sun glasses. The Polar bear also sits in the sun shielding its eyes with a front paw.

Owls use their third eyelids as transparent windows to shade the eyes from daylight, while many migratory birds it is thought close their third eyelids during their long flights.

The third eyelid, in most animals which possess it, is operated when the eye is automatically drawn back into the orbit by contraction of the retractor muscle of the eye. This takes place whenever a speck of dust falls upon the eye, or when the animal fears violence, or that the sensitive eyeball may be likely to be touched. The postorbital fat is intended to act as a buffer to protect the eyeball, but the fat is attached also to the base of the third eyelid. When the eye retracts and presses upon the fat, this moves sideways up the eyeball and pushes the third eyelid upwards to partly cover the eye.

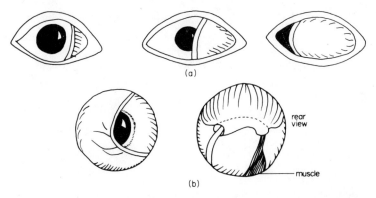

Fig. 3 The membrana nictitans (third eyelid).
    (a)   Mammalian type as in cat and dog, showing three stages of closure.
    (b)   In the birds. Unlike the mammals, there is no retractor muscle.

Birds, frogs, alligators and turtles all possess a third eyelid, but they have no retractor eye muscle and so the pull upon the third eyelid or nictitating membrane, is exerted through a muscle and its tendon. The latter passes through a pulley-like loop at the back of the eye and in this way is able to draw the third eyelid directly over the front of the eyeball.

When we wonder how well or how much any animal can see, we must allow for several features, not universally common:

(1) *The distance of the head from the ground.* A giraffe can look through the treetops. A rat has eyes close to the ground.

(2) *The position of the eyes in the head;* whether they are placed frontally, as in the cat and some of the short-faced Toy dogs, or *almost* frontally as in the Toy Poodle and Maltese Terrier. In birds and fishes the eyes are usually on either side of the head. In the larger

breeds of dogs the eyes are placed at an angle of 30–35 degrees from the mid-line of the forehead, so that the two eyes cannot *converge* upon a distant object, which can be seen with only one eye at a time. Some eyes have large open pupils, particularly when the

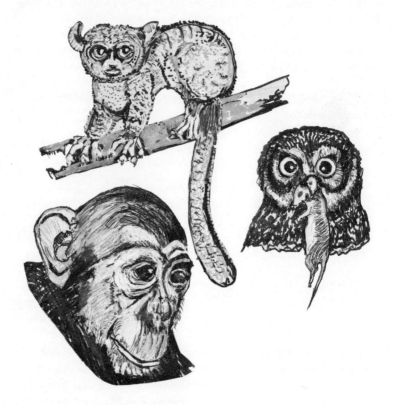

Fig. 4   Frontal vision in various animals: Bushbaby; Little Owl; Chimpanzee.

owner is excited or moving rapidly, and it is more difficult to focus an object lying ahead with an open pupil than with one which is contracted to provide only a small aperture.

(3) *The size and width of the head between the eyes.* As we shall find later, a horse cannot see past its own brow and muzzle when the eyes are directed downward. When approaching a jump, its vision ceases four feet from the obstacle.

(4) *The amount of eye movement possible.* In an owl the eyes are fixed and devoid of movement, but to compensate for this the neck is extremely flexible, so that the owl can actually turn its head upside down.

(5) *The degree of neck movement possible.* This varies immensely even in dogs. Many animals find it far easier to move the head and neck than the eyes. Snakes use head movements in every direction. Whales have massive eye muscles but never use them. The elephant has little or no eye movement.

(6) *The degree by which the eyes protrude from the eyelids,* (proptosis), may determine the degree of vision possible. A Fox terrier shows little of the eye and a Pekinese shows a large amount of eye. In these two breeds the actual size of whole eye is very similar.

(7) *The quality of the retina.* The ability to focus (convergence), and the capability of the animal's brain to make use of available information all play an important part in producing the visual impression, and making use of it to the best advantage.

(8) Photographers speak of cameras as having a 'wide-angle' lens which takes in a considerable 'field' in each exposure; whereas another camera may cover only a very narrow area. Some animals have a wider view than others because their eyes are laterally placed and between them they cover two separate viewpoints, each of which may be fairly wide. The ox does this but may fail to see objects directly ahead. This is one reason why bullfighters have a better expectation of life than snake-charmers. Nevertheless, a cow can often see its flanks, and can kick forwards. This is a fact well known to every person who milks cows! A hare can actually see behind it and keep a jump ahead of the greyhound attempting to grab hold of it. Unfortunately, however, whilst thus occupied it sees little of what lies ahead and can easily come into collision; or as has been known, it may gallop over a cliff while keeping its eyes fixed on the space behind it.

DISTANCE PERCEPTION IN OTHER ANIMALS COMPARED WITH MAMMALS

The bat living in a constant state of near-blindness, depends upon its own radar, making use of supersonic vibrations issuing through nose or mouth, while it registers the echoes rebounding from obstacles in front. Gannets pick out a fish from a shoal, or, from a high place in the sky observe a shoal and drop like stones. The Kingfisher, in one lightning-like flash, can dive under water from a bough, spear a fish, and be back upon the bough in a few seconds.

The chameleon, sluggish in movement, can thrust out an enormously long tongue and collect a fly without fail. An Archer fish can see a fly hovering about eighteen inches above the surface of the water, spit a jet of water at it, and bring it to the surface ready to be collected.

In animals, movement perception is of great importance. A dog may watch the surface of a field from a distance for several minutes and see nothing. But when a rabbit, formerly still and invisible, makes a move, the distance between the rabbit and some neighbour-ing fixed object changes and the dog immediately springs into action. And yet few dogs, cats or other animals apart perhaps from an occasional monkey, recognise other animals on a television screen or watch their movements with any interest, particularly if the sound is turned off.

The eyes are protected and saved from becoming dry by blinking. In different animals the rate of blinking varies from 8–12 blinks a minute. This applies also to human eyes. In some animals blinking is performed less frequently—this applies to the dog. This is in marked contrast to what happens in birds, which often blink so rapidly and so frequently that the movement can scarcely be detected.

PARALLAX AND PARALLACTIC DISPLACEMENT

When a human head is moved from side to side, objects near the observer, seem to move (in relation to more distant objects) in the opposite direction. If the observer takes a step forward the objects nearest to his eyes appear to move past him while more distant objects move with him. When at rest in a secluded spot, the view may occasionally appear to be quite motionless, but directly the head is set in motion, the whole landscape or environment appears to spring to life on account of parallactic displacements. This is because of the three-dimensional nature of the image reaching the retina. Parallax and parallactic displacement is more obvious in the Primates provided with full frontal vision than it is in animals such as the horse and ox, and in certain breeds of dogs, in which the forehead is wide between the eyes, and the eyes themselves are set more or less obliquely and at an angle with the midline of the face and forehead. In the horse and ox, to take examples of a vast number of wide-browed animals, the eyeball tends to retain a horizontal position so that, whatever the position of the head, the line of vision remains parallel with the ground.

EYE MOVEMENTS

In the majority of animals below the Primates in the social scale, eye movements are secondary to head movements. There would be no advantage in most animals, provided with necks of reasonable length, to devote too much space in the orbit to the development of muscles to operate eye movements, when the head can be swung into the required position almost instantaneously and brought to a standstill.

The only animals which need a great deal of ability to move the eyes in the orbit are those possessing a superior type of retina with an area centralis, a fovea or centre of supreme sensitivity, packed with cones to provide a marked acuity of vision.

Even birds and reptiles which possess foveae seldom make great use of the oculo-motor muscles they may possess. They too, have very flexible necks. It is doubtful even whether Man would have required such development of eye muscles and an area centralis, if he had been provided with a more swan-like neck. In any case, even we ourselves, see very little while our neck or our eyes are moving. We can study detail only when our eyes are stationary and focussed upon the object requiring examination. People reading a page of moderate width, say four inches of type, may move their heads slightly from side to side; others keep the head still and employ their wide angle of vision to take it all in. We do this more so when viewing a small picture than when reading print, every word of which may have meaning. The only people who did this regularly were accountants, but that was before the days of the adding machine. Animals tend to carry their eyes in the horizontal position whatever the position of the head. Dogs seldom lift their eyes, even when the head is held firmly. In mammals which have any pretence to eye movement, the two eyes work in conjunction but in bats, rats, mice, rabbits, and in some insectivorous animals, the two eyes are often capable of working singly.

The power to make use of binocular vision, with convergence and accommodation (the power of focusing) is present in the Primates, including human children, at quite an early age. If we place a dog

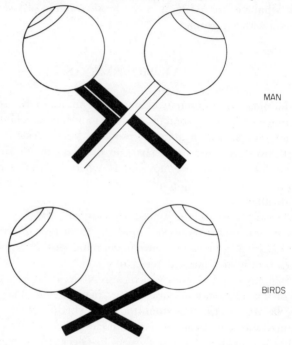

MAN

BIRDS

Fig. 5   The optic nerve and its decussation. In animals such as man, half the optic nerve fibres go to the same side of the brain and half to the other side. This makes stereoscopic vision possible. In animals in which the eyes are laterally placed, far fewer fibres go to the side on which the eye is situated. In birds all the fibres cross to the opposite side of the brain.

on a table and persuade it to look straight ahead and we then draw an imaginary line through the plane of the right eye and another through the plane of the left eye, we can imagine these lines meeting behind the dog's head. The angle at which these lines meet will be the dog's 'visual angle'. The visual angles in Terriers is usually from 18–25 degrees as compared with 5–10 degrees in Pekinese.

In the cat the angle is 8–18 degrees.

In Man it is nil.

In order to possess good stereoscopic vision, binocular vision is indispensable. The second cranial nerve is the optic nerve which passes through the optic foramen in the skull, behind the eyeball and enters the eye at the optic papilla. Nerve fibres from the retina, converge at the optic papilla and leave the eye within the optic nerve, which passes through the foramen on its way to the brain.

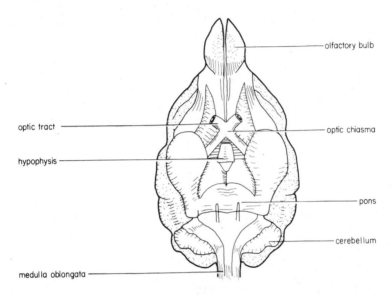

Fig. 6 Base of the brain of the dog showing the optic tract and the optic chiasma.

The optic nerve is thick and round. The fibres of either side cross each other in close adhesion, at the base of the brain. Some of the fibres from one nerve may cross over to the other side of the chiasma and return to the brain in the opposite tract. This decussation (crossing) of nerve fibres is essential to stereoscopic vision, in which the three dimensions of space are observed at the same time.

In man and the Primates, stereoscopic vision is good; in the cats in which there is only a slight divergence of the optic axis, it is quite good. In the dog it varies according to the breed.

In those breeds with frontal eye placement and binocular vision the degree of stereoscopic vision equals that of the cat. As the degree of binocular vision increases, the eyes converge less, the visual fields

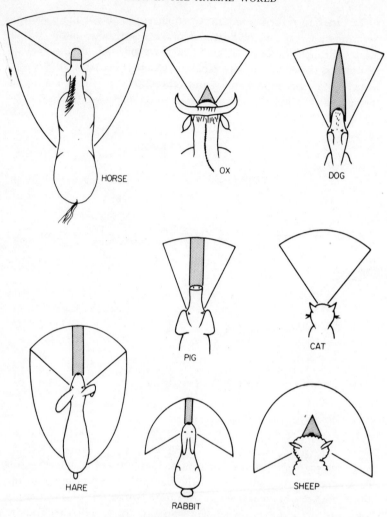

Fig. 7   The limits of binocular vision in various animals. The shading in front indicates the 'blind' areas.

tend to overlap, and so straight paths begin to merge with decussating fibres and stereoscopic vision becomes established. In birds, fishes and some of the lower vertebrates, the optic fibres cross completely, with perception of sensation transmitted to the opposite cerebral lobe of the brain. In animals in which the eyes are on opposite sides of the head instead of being frontally directed, crossing is complete. Stereoscopic vision relates to the ability to visualise an object as a solid. To do this each eye must see the object in such a way that it acquires a particular similarity and a particular dissimilarity on the impression received by each retina, the degree of eye convergence producing retinal images of the right kind in the right place. The two retinal views must be opposites; one must be a right-handed and the other a left-handed representation of the same object. If the two pictures do not overlap, or tally properly, they cannot terminate in a single image and confusion must result.

The popular view is that true stereoscopic vision can be achieved only when *all* the fibres do not cross over to the opposite side of the brain, but a certain proportion of the fibres pass to the same side of the brain. In the dog one quarter of the fibres travel to the same side of the brain and three quarters decussate. In the cat one third go to the same side. In the horse one sixth to one eighth of the nerve fibres go to the same side; in the rat and opossum, one fifth. In animals with completely binocular vision the number remaining on the same side is very small. The rabbit is something of an exception because it has eyes laterally placed and yet has some fibres which do not cross. Fishes have none which do not cross.

COLOUR VISION

Colour vision is denied to dogs and cats because the rods and cones in their retinae are unable to discriminate. But the apes and monkeys (some of them); birds, and some kinds of fishes, see colours. So do quite a number of insects, but the elephants and camels and the beasts of prey, the hippopotamus and the rhinoceros, have no sense of colour at all.

Birds recognise their mates and their companions by the colour of their plumage. Some, such as the Bower bird, appear to exhibit aesthetic appreciation when they select bright articles and coloured ones to incorporate in their nests. Among some varieties of birds the retinae have long slender cones containing droplets of oil, varying in colour from red to orange and from yellow to pale green. These affect the colour sensitivity of birds. The droplets act as filters, restricting the amount of blue light reaching the sensitive limbs of the cones. This gives improved visibility of distant objects. It may enable a hawk, flying high in the air to see the mouse on the soil below. Oil droplets are also present in the retinae of frogs, lizards, turtles and a great many reptiles.

Anglers all maintain that slight variation in the shade of an artificial fly may make all the difference to the weight of their catch. It is unlikely that a fish in water can recognise colours in a *dry* fly floating on the surface of the water, feet above its head. It is likely, however, that a *wet* coloured fly can be recognised by many varieties of fish. Some are attracted by brightness rather than by colour.

Bleak, sticklebacks and some other fish, prefer blue or red, to green. Others select blue or red baits, but seldom both. Many can show their preference for red worms, or red rag. Roach favour red or yellow-dyed maggots. The cartilaginous fishes, including the sharks, dog fish and rays, are quite unable to decide between colours.

Bees are believed to favour flowers of particular colours, and wasps and butterflies are credited with colour vision. There is, however, a possibility that these insects may be attracted more by scent than by vision. Moths are attracted by bright colours and bright lights, but the attraction is believed to be from brightness rather than colour.

Caterpillars usually prefer plants whose colours camouflage them. It is unlikely that they choose their environment by the aid of a colour sense. It is possible that those which favoured certain plants survived, while those which favoured other contrasting plants, died out. The survival of the fortunate feeders may have been brought about in this way.

DAY AND NIGHT VISION

Diurnal animals move about in daylight; nocturnal animals normally move about in darkness. Arhythmic animals sleep by day or by night, and walk about when they are awake. The Prairie Dog, the accepted example of the arhythmic type, needs to be able to see in the dark as well as in daylight. It has a yellow lens which may in some way assist in this facility. Dogs, rats, cats and a variety of other animals possess a tapetum. This is a glistening opaque layer underlying the retina in place of the deeply pigmented choroid coat. It reflects light back through the retina and increases the power of perception. In some plates and films employed in photography, a similar backing is used to improve the picture taken in a dim light. In animals

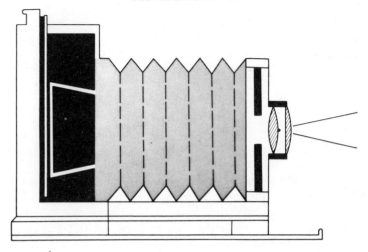

Fig. 8 The camera and the eye. The diagram represents a
section of a simple camera. Rays of light pass through a
compound lens (equivalent to the cornea and optic lens of the
eye) and fall upon a light-sensitive surface at the back of the
eye, the sensitive plate or film, (equivalent to the retina of the
eye). In both camera and eye the light rays pass through an
adjustable diaphragm (the iris of the eye). The hinder surface of
the film is protected from light by the black paper in which the
film is rolled; in the eye the choroid coat underlies the retina and
performs this function.

In some animals an iridescent tapetum reflects some of the light
rays back through the retina. In some manufactured films and
plates a backing of a mirror-like substance performs the same
purpose.

Focusing is carried out in the camera by moving the lens
nearer or farther away from the light-sensitive film. In the eye
this is also done by some animals (fishes); in others the lens
increases or diminishes its curvature.

In the camera, providing there is ample lighting, the necessity
for very accurate focusing can be lessened by reducing the size of
the aperture of the diaphragm. Many animals make use of this
'pinhole' method in bright sunlight.

provided with a tapetum, light may be reflected back from the
glistening surface. It is possible by shining a torch, or the headlights
of a car, into eyes during darkness to determine which animals have
a tapetum. Man is not provided for in this way, but in people sitting
round a camp fire, human eyes will glow with a reddish tint.
However, this is due to the circulating blood in the vessels within

the retina. One of the most useful adjuncts to the eye, required for use in darkness, is a pupil which will dilate widely within a short time of exposure to a dim light.

NIGHT BLINDNESS

A certain number of animals see well only during the hours of daylight, while others probably see better during the hours of darkness; this may bear a relationship to the ability of the pupil to dilate more fully in conditions of darkness provided there is a little illumination from the moon or stars. Such animals may see even better than the animals they hunt. A third type, the arhythmic animal, sees fairly well in the dim light of dawn and dusk and prefers to sleep or seek cover during the hours of bright daylight or the darkness of night.

But animals which normally see fairly well in both daylight and in dim light may develop a form of night blindness which may be associated either with lack of vitamin A in their diet, or with inability to make use of the supply available. There is also a form of night blindness which is recognised frequently nowadays, particularly in dogs, and is regarded as hereditary. It may appear at any time during the first few years of life and is progressive in character. It is due to atrophy of the retina arising from gradual degeneration (and ultimate disappearance) of the blood vessels which normally radiate over the surface of the retina and provide it with nourishment.

CHAPTER 3

THE HUMAN EYE

The human eye is typical of the mammalian eye in general, although variations occur in many species. In man, the eyes lie beneath the level of the brows. Each is contained within a rounded cavity in the

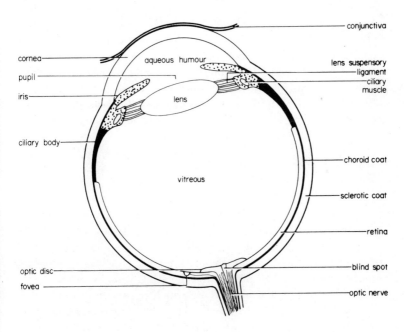

Fig. 9   Section of the human eye.

skull, known as the orbit, with the nasal bones lying between them. The eyeball is practically spherical and resembles a globe from which a fifth part of the circumference is missing. Into the aperture is fitted a clear but slightly smaller segment.

31

To appreciate this arrangement better, take paper and a pair of compasses. Open out the compasses until the lead of the pencil and the sharp point of the compass are about an inch apart. Now draw an arc roughly representing four-fifths of the entire surface, leaving the gap on the left side of the paper. Now move the sharp point of the compass horizontally a quarter of an inch to the left, and again insert it in the paper. Adjust the position of the pencil point until the lead makes contact with one end of the arc you previously made. Rotate the compass until the pencil fills the gap in the original larger arc. The second, and smaller arc, will now protrude a little out of line with the larger one. The protruding portion represents the transparent cornea in front of the eye. The larger portion is the eyeball proper.

In man, a little more than half the eyeball is contained within the bony circle of the orbit, while the remainder of the eyeball protrudes outside the orbit, well covered, however, by large, mobile eyelids, an upper and a lower. These carry the eyelashes: longer on the upper lids than upon the lower. They are very efficient at keeping dust and grit from falling upon and damaging the very sensitive cornea. Man lacks the third eyelid which is present in a large proportion of the world's mammals. This lies beneath the main eyelids and sweeps over the cornea after the manner of a car's screenwiper.

THE LID-CLOSURE REFLEX

In man this reflex protects the eye against any visible possibility of injury by instantaneous closure of the lids. It is associated with a contraction of the pupil. The eyeball is protected against external pressure and forcible injury by the presence of a large pad of fat upon which the eyeball rests within the orbit: its bony casing.

Most mammals, and all of those which possess the third eyelid, also have a muscle, known as the retractor muscle of the eyeball, which draws the eyeball backward into the socket formed by the orbit when injury threatens. At the same time, the withdrawal of the eye into the orbit sets in motion the reflex which lifts the third eyelid up and over the cornea.

Man lacks this retractor muscle, as well as the third eyelid, and is therefore compelled to depend upon either a reflex or a voluntary closing of the eyelids (providing the approaching object can be seen and recognised). Actual closing of the eyelids may protect the sensitive cornea but this may be insufficient to save the deeper parts of the eyeball from injury. Man is therefore entirely dependent against a more substantial eye injury, upon the pad of fat behind the eyeball into which the whole structure will be forced. When we consider the more elaborate mechanism provided for other mammals, provided also with the third eyelid and the retractor muscle, we may feel some surprise that man is not better equipped in this respect.

Although man is not provided with horns, he is still in danger from animals which do possess them. Man's defence before he discovered the use of weapons, could only have been his fists, and the human eyeball can sustain serious injury from uncovered knuckles.

THE CONJUNCTIVA

This is a moist, sensitive membrane which forms a continuous covering over the inner surface of the eyelids and the outer surface of the eyeball. It is specially modified where it covers the cornea. Since the membrane is continuous from the inside of the lids and over the eyeball it forms a pouch which is called the *conjunctival sac*. The portion overlying the cornea is extremely sensitive, the remainder less so. The whole of the outer surface of the eyeball, with the exception of the transparent cornea, is made up of a tough grey tunic known as the sclera, or sclerotic membrane. The front portion of this membrane is missing and into the aperture is fitted the cornea, overlapping the sclera very slightly just like a watch glass lying on the front surface of a watch.

The next layer of the outer covering of the eyeball, lying immediately under the sclera, is black, and is known as the choroid coat or membrane (see later). The purpose of this deeply pigmented lining is to prevent loss of light, or scattering of the light rays which are destined to alight upon the inner surface of the retina. The retina is a thin membrane—in spite of the fact that it is made up of about ten layers of cells, all different, many of them being nerve cells. In shape it resembles that of a saucer with the concave surface facing forwards so that every portion is equidistant from the lens. This ensures that every part of the picture upon the retina is in focus.

Light enters the eye through the cornea and then through the pupil of the iris. In man, the pupil is a round opening of variable diameter passing through the centre of the iris. The iris is a pigmented (except in albinos) membranous structure containing both circular and radial muscular fibres stretching across the anterior chamber of the eye between the inner surface of the cornea and the crystalline lens of the eye. When the light is dim the radial muscular fibres in the iris contract and increase the diameter of the pupil.

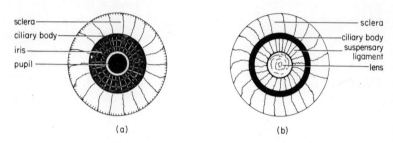

(a)   (b)

Fig. 10   (a)   Front of human eye with eyelids removed.
          (b)   Front of eye with cornea removed.
          (From Thomson Henderson's collection.)

When the light is bright the circular muscle fibres come into action and the diameter of the iris aperture diminishes. As the intensity of light varies almost constantly, the size of the aperture of the pupil keeps changing quite automatically. If one shuts an eye for a few moments, thus cutting out the light, the pupil dilates, and can be seen to be contracting as soon as the eye is opened and again receiving the light rays. After travelling through the pupil of the eye the rays of light pass through the biconvex crystalline lens. The rays then converge and land upon the surface of the retina, upon which they form an image. One would be surprised, if one could see it, how very small the image is, and, of course, upside down. The image is picked up by the fibres of the optic nerve within the retina and conveyed to the appropriate portion of the brain.

This is all brought about by stimulation of nerve cells in the substance of the retina by light rays. If one stimulates these same nerve cells, not by light rays but by any other form of stimulation, such as pressing upon the eyeball for a few seconds with the ball of the finger, one may 'see' light. After more severe stimulation as by a blow, the owner of the eye may 'see stars' which is another example of the impression of light derived from a more active form of stimulation. As soon as the tension of the suspensory ligament is withdrawn the lens, being elastic, resumes its normal contour.

This may seem a very extraordinary method of obtaining a correct focus but the only other way in which this could have been effected would have been by introducing some way of moving the lens slightly forward and backward. This would have been a difficult process and in reality the method adopted appears to be not only very ingenious but also very effective. When we consider the means of focussing adopted in other species we shall find a number of other methods, specially adapted to the animal and its environment.

The ability to obtain a correct focus at will, is termed 'the power of accommodation'. In actual fact, focussing the eye upon an object is not quite as simple as it might appear to be. In mammals the cornea is slightly convex on its anterior surface and the anterior chamber of the eyeball is filled with a clear saline fluid. The cornea is devoid of blood vessels and is perfectly clear and transparent. The combination of the convex cornea and the fluid lying in front of the lens of the eye, together constitute a magnifying lens. This combines with the true crystalline lens of the eye to form a compound lens. The distance the light rays have to travel through the clear jelly-like vitreous humour which fills the posterior chamber of the eye is approximately 8 mm, so the degree of adjustment required to obtain the correct focus is not so very great.

The human eye in many ways resembles some of the modern types of box camera in which the distance between lens and sensitive film is equally short and within certain limits focussing is dispensed with. In the older cameras which employed bellows to move the lens forward or backward, the focal length might have been anything up to about ten inches. One marked difference between the eye and the camera lies in the amount of time between exposure and development of the picture. The photographic film has to be developed and printed but the retinal image is carried to the brain instantly, and the interval between focussing an object and perceiving it is negligible. One feature common to the eye and the camera is the necessity to vary the amount of light admitted through the lens by the use of a diaphragm with a variable aperture. In the eyes of mammals this is effected by the use of the pupil of the iris which adjusts itself to the degree of illumination at any given moment.

Some of the modern cameras copy this by being provided with

an automatic adjustment which varies the aperture in accordance with the degree of light present at the time.

The whole of the interior of the eye, apart from the space occupied by the transparent cornea, is lined by the choroid, which is black, and the interior of the camera is similarly protected, while the film itself is lined with black paper. In some animals other than man, instead of the completely black layer lying behind the retina (the choroid), a brighter reflecting surface is interposed. The purpose of this is to reflect some of the light falling upon the surface of the retina back again so as to produce a double exposure. The layer which glistens in this way is termed the tapetum and as one might expect, it is found in those animals which wander and hunt by night when there is a minimum amount of light available.

Eyes are termed diurnal when they function better in daytime, and nocturnal when they come into use more efficiently during the hours of darkness. In some animals such as those of the cat family, the eyes are adapted to function equally well by day and by night, and the tapetum is mainly concerned in bringing this about. Some dogs exhibit eyeshine by night, but not all. The human eye is able to 'see' a considerable number of separate pictures in the space of a second and recognise from them what we regard as 'movement'. Movement perception is probably much less important to man than to other animals, apart from the fact that he is exposed more frequently to traffic hazards. However, mankind becomes more or less educated in dealing with such risks, whereas animals, lower in the evolutionary scale, seldom grasp the fact that vehicles may travel faster than they themselves can do. In this way they create unnecessary hazards and pay the cost.

. Much depends upon whether the animal possesses binocular or only monocular vision: in other words, whether the shape of its head enables it to look straight ahead with two eyes at a time or only with one eye. Intelligent animals with binocular vision are able to use their judgement and maintain what they regard as a safe 'escape distance'. Some other animals may not accept such ideas. Mice, for instance, wait for nothing and bolt as soon as they sense danger— which is at least, one reason why there are so many mice!

Another factor which contributes to our own safety is that many moving objects produce a recognisable sound and many of the projectiles (apart from bullets) which we dread most, are now provided with instruments calculated to give audible notice of their approach. We are enabled, therefore, in many instances to make use of two senses simultaneously.

The orbit in man, as previously stated, protects the eye from injury from without, while the lids and their lashes bend to prevent foreign bodies or dust falling upon the sensitive cornea. In addition the eyelids respond rapidly to the mildest stimulus and close whenever danger threatens. The lids blink at intervals and so act in the manner of screenwipers, while a flow of tears from the lachrymal gland enters the eye and escapes through the lachrymal duct at the anterior corner of the eye, to run down into the nostrils. This stream helps to remove dust particles as well as any irritants which may accidentally enter the lachrymal sac (the space between the eye and the eyeball, enclosed in conjunctiva).

In some animals such as birds, fishes and reptiles in which the aperture between the eyelids (the palpebral orifice) is small, the eyeball is relatively larger than it is in man and most other mammals. The reason is that in these other animals as much as three-quarters of the eyeball is concealed within the orbit.

In man, who operates mainly during the hours of daylight (or did so before artificial lighting was invented) the cornea occupies only seventeen per cent of the total globe area; in nocturnal animals it occupies up to thirty-five per cent. The lens is held in place by the suspensory ligament, also known as the zonule. This consists of radial strands of the tough fibrous protein, collagen. One end of the zonular fibres is attached to the lens capsule at the equator while the other is adherent to the ciliary body (described later). This structural arrangement plays a great part in focussing the retinal image.

Although the lens appears quite homogenuous to the human eye, its internal structure as revealed in microscopical sections, is, in fact, quite complex. Briefly, it consists of a nucleus, surrounded by the cortex. The anterior layer is covered by a single layer of cuboidal cells: the lens epithelium. The remainder of the lens is made up of narrow elongated cells: the lens fibres. These run in an anterior–posterior direction and are packed closely together. New lens fibres develop throughout life so that the lens never stops growing. New fibres are produced at the lens equator where epithelial cells elongate into fibres. The epithelial cells used up in this way are replaced by cell division elsewhere in the epithelium, so that the epithelium has to grow in order to keep pace with the fibres. Since new fibres are constantly being added onto the outside of the existing fibres, the oldest fibres in any lens will always be in the middle portion with the youngest fibres nearest the outside. The lens substance consists entirely of lens fibres and epithelium, without blood vessels or nerves.

The lens throws off its worn cells but as these cannot pass through the capsule, they cannot escape. Consequently, the lens goes on growing all its life. Between 0 and 9 years it weighs approximately 130 mg but at about 80–90, it weighs 255 mg. As a result of growth, the curvature of the outer zone decreases and the lens gets much flatter, but as the refractive power of the lens nucleus increases, the effect on vision is less than might be expected. When the lens does not compensate in this way, the eye becomes hypermetropic or long-sighted. In early cataract, the lens nucleus hardens and the eye becomes myopic or shortsighted.

ACCOMMODATION

The lens is kept in place, behind the iris, by means of a ligament known as the suspensory ligament, which is attached around its circumference and along its upper edge to the ciliary processes, which are a continuation of the black choroid coat extending almost to the outer circumference of the cornea.

This ligament is made up of minute, rope-like strands of tissue. The ciliary processes to which these strands are attached carry in their substance a muscle termed the ciliary muscle. When an attempt is made to focus the eye upon an object, the ciliary muscle contracts just sufficiently, and in so doing it tightens the suspensory fibres and exerts a pull upon the circumference of the lens. This tightens the lens capsule, squeezes the elastic lens and causes its bulging surfaces to flatten. By reducing its curvature it alters and corrects the focus.

THE CORNEA

The cornea is the anterior portion of the globe of the eye, completely transparent and sometimes referred to as 'the window of the eye'.

It is tough but its thickness varies with its topography. The normal average thickness of the human cornea is 0·5 mm at the centre and 1 mm at its periphery. It is faintly elastic. The cornea contains no blood vessels unless as the result of injury or inflammatory changes.

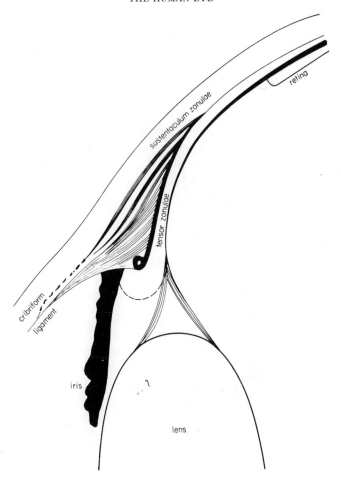

Fig. 11(*a*)   The human eye in static position (After Thomson
Henderson).

It obtains most of its metabolic needs through the aqueous humour
via the endothelium. During waking hours the cornea absorbs some
oxygen from the air and when covered by the eyelids derives it from
the neighbouring bloodstream, having no blood vessels of its own. It
is dependent for its wellbeing upon a sufficiency of vitamin A, a
deficiency of which causes it to become dull, thickened and cloudy.

C

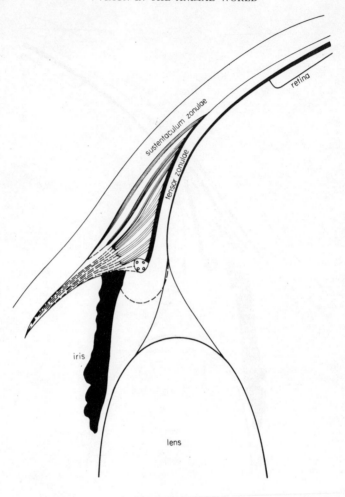

Fig. 11(*b*) The human eye in active accommodation (After
Thomson Henderson).

The cornea is composed of five layers:
From the outside, these are:
(*a*) Epithelium, comprising surface, wing and basal cells.
(*b*) Bowman's membrane. Thin, particularly so in the lower
orders of mammals, somewhat elastic.

(c) The *substantia propria* (stroma). The cornea is composed of plates and bundles of lamellae composed of collagen, alternating at right angles. The union between successive layers is not intimate with the result that lymph spaces remain. In addition to lymph, these spaces

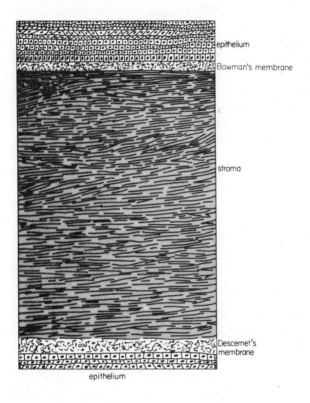

Fig. 12 Section through the human cornea.

contain corneal corpuscles, corpuscular in the horse and ox; membranous in the dog and in man. The others consist of wandering white corpuscles (leucocytes) which have escaped from the surrounding blood vessels of the limbus, or from neighbouring capillaries. Most of these corpuscles are possessed of long protoplasmic threads or branches. These are linked up so that nutrient materials, as well as waste products, can be carried to and from the marginal cells.

In addition to corneal corpuscles and leucocytes, the stroma (substantia propria), contains cells known as keratocytes which manufacture collagen.

(d) Descemet's membrane

This is a thick, homogeneous, hyaloid and very elastic membrane deposited by the epithelial cells lining the posterior surface of the cornea. The degree of elasticity is so marked that the membrane is enabled to bulge through any breach arising in the substantia propria, and maintain the continuity of the anterior chamber for long periods (as during corneal ulceration), without any loss of aqueous humour. The membrane is about 5 microns thick in the foal but its thickness increases in all animals with advancing age. Thus, in an aged horse the membrane may be 0·1 mm in thickness. When it becomes torn, or when it eventually bursts in a case of corneal ulceration, it never regenerates or heals, but the gap becomes plugged by an ingrowth of endothelial cells which creep into the rent.

(e) Posterior endothelium (epithelium)

This lines the cornea and is composed of a layer of flattened polygonal cells, which line Descemet's membrane and help to maintain it while at the same time providing a waterproofing barrier, and protecting the cornea from direct contact with the aqueous humour. This membrane is continuous with the anterior covering of the iris.

The posterior wall of the cornea forms the anterior boundary of the chamber which contains the aqueous humour. The curvature of the cornea is less than that of the sclerotic so that, viewing the eyeball as a whole (as in a post-mortem specimen), the cornea appears flatter than the remainder of the eyeball. In such a specimen there may be obvious shrinkage owing to draining away of some of the aqueous fluid into the spaces of Fontana (especially in the human eye) and also into the suprachoroidal space (especially in the dog and lower orders of mammals).

AQUEOUS HUMOUR

The aqueous humour is a saline fluid and it occupies that portion of the eyeball bounded by the anterior surface of the lens and the posterior layer of the cornea. This fluid has very specific constituents and is continually being synthesised and removed. Excessive production of the fluid, or any breakdown in the mechanism responsible for its removal, may result in a change in the corneal curvature. This is especially evident in the condition known as glaucoma.

Glaucoma is common in man but less so in the dog, for example. The reason is that man is mainly dependent for its removal upon the canal of Schlemm which may become partially occluded by any abnormality arising in the angle of filtration. The raising of intra-ocular pressure in animals other than man, and mammals in particular, produces not a glaucoma but a bulging of the cornea as a result of the retina and choroid coats being pushed tightly up against the sclera with a resulting obliteration of the suprachoroidal space. This enlargement of the eyeball is termed hydrophthalmos. Among some of the lower orders there would appear to be no very reliable provision made by the interior of the eye for the rapid changing of fluids.

The aqueous fluid is secreted by the epithelium of the ciliary processes and in animals such as man, who possess a functioning canal of Schlemm, the intraocular pressure is balanced by the pressure existing in the veins as they pass out of the eyeball. In the lower orders, at least, the exit of the aqueous into the lymphatic spaces, via the suprachoroidal space, maintains pressure equilibrium. After the fluid has emerged from the capillaries of the ciliary epithelium it is believed, in the higher animals, to enter the posterior chamber. When this chamber is poorly developed as in Herbivora and Carnivora, the fluid passes between the suspensory ligament and the posterior surface of the iris and reaches the anterior chamber by passing through the pupillary opening.

The movement of the aqueous humour into and out of the anterior chamber is continuous and more rapid than might be imagined. Various measures have been devised to ascertain the rate of flow. One method is by ascertaining how quickly water, containing heavy hydrogen in the molecule, appears in the aqueous humour after it has been injected into some other part of the animal body. By this means it is possible to determine the volume of this substance which reaches the aqueous humour within a given time as well as the interval which elapses while the exchange of the material takes place between the blood and the aqueous fluid. In experiments conducted in this way with rabbits, it has been estimated that one half of the aqueous content of the anterior chamber is exchanged every three minutes. This result may be a little misleading because it probably takes longer to exchange solids in solution than to transfer plain water. Nevertheless, it indicates that the rate of exchange is fairly rapid. In surgical operations, when the anterior chamber has been drained as during lens extraction, refilling of the sutured chamber is completed within two or three hours.

It must, however, be admitted that in such cases there may already be some existing obstruction to the outflow of fluid from the anterior chamber back into the circulation.

Davson, in *Physiology of the Eye*, states: 'When aqueous humour is withdrawn from the eye in appreciable quantities, the fluid is reformed rapidly, but is now no longer normal, the concentration of proteins being raised.' Estimates on the principle of using a marker agree on a value of some 1 to $1\frac{1}{2}$ per cent of the total volume per minute. Thus, in the cat, with a total volume of about 1 ml, this would correspond to 10–15 μl/min, whilst in the rabbit, with a volume of about 0·35 ml, the absolute flow rate would be less, namely 3·5–5·2 μl/min.

THE SCLEROTIC COAT OR SCLERA

The sclera is a strong, opaque fibrous membrane composed of connective tissue containing a large number of white fibres and a small number of fine elastic fibres.

It is made up of four layers:

 (*a*) tenons capsule
 (*b*) episcleral tissue
 (*c*) sclera proper
 (*d*) lamina fusca

It is continuous with the cornea at its limbus. The bundles of fibres are disposed meridianally and equatorially, and beneath the surface have a felted arrangement, whereas the surface fibres are arranged in a longitudinal manner. The sclera not only maintains the shape of the eyeball but also controls the intraorbital pressure and protects the vascular tissues lying immediately beneath it within its wall. It covers the eyeball except for the portion covered by the cornea, which it overlaps at its rim in the fashion of the metal case of a watch enclosing a glass. The sclera is thick at its rim but becomes thinner immediately external to it so that the underlying pigmented choroid, lying immediately beneath it, may impart a bluish tint in the human eye, to the visible portion of the 'white of the eye'. The pressure within the blood vessels of the sclera is normally low and in health they will probably remain invisible unless some inflammatory condition supervenes, when they may become congested and plainly visible.

In the domesticated animals the sclera is less resistant to internal pressure and a lowered calcium level may further reduce its strength. Whereas in man a simple glaucoma may exist; in the dog, cat, horse or ox, a hydrophthalmus may make its appearance. This, however, reduces the pressure upon the optic disc as compared with glaucoma. In its hinder half the sclera thickens a great deal, especially where it encases the optic nerve. This emerges from the eyeball, a little below and slightly lateral to its centre. The nerve bundles separate out here and pass through a number of small apertures in the choroid coat which lies beneath the sclera. This sieve-like area is known as the lamina cribrosa. In man it is well developed but in other animals, outside some of the Primates, it is not so well marked and is represented by the choroidal portion only.

The muscles which control eye movement are inserted into the more anterior part of the scleral wall. Present in man, but particularly well developed in the lower species, is a lymph space lying between the scleral and choroid coats. This has received the titles perichoroidal and/or suprachoroidal space. It arises from bifurcation of the cribriform ligament and is a continuation of the spaces contained within this structure. The space contains a quantity of loose pigmented connective tissue which, being porous, permits through it the passage of aqueous humour into the venous plexus situated in that region. Between the scleral and choroid coats, and within the suprachoroidal space, a number of connective tissue projections appear, and these interweave sufficiently to hold the two coats in position with enough intervening space to permit the passage of fluids. The rigidity of the scleral coat is essential to accommodation, since accurate focussing for the purpose of visual definition demands that the length of the eyeball from cornea to retina shall remain constant. Without scleral rigidity the squeezing effect of the eyelids and the intraorbital muscles would result in lengthening of the eyeball. In some species of vertebrates this difficulty is overcome by a reinforcement of bone or cartilage.

THE CHOROID COAT

This is a vascular, black or dark brown basin-shaped membrane which lines the sclerotic coat and comes between it and the retina. Its purpose is to cause rays of light to impinge upon the retina without unnecessary wastage. It corresponds with the black sheet placed behind the film in the camera. In addition it carries large blood vessels and a rich network of capillaries. Between it and the sclera exist the suprachoroidal spaces through which, particularly in the lower orders of mammals, aqueous humour is drawn off into the lymph channels.

MOVEMENTS OF THE EYEBALL

In man the movements of the eyeball are very free in every direction, except laterally. He raises his eyes aloft with ease whereas most animals make use of the neck and lift the head. In a great many animals the pupils remain vertical in whatever position the head is held.

In man six muscles are connected with the eyeball, four straight and two oblique. The straight muscles (recti) pull the eyes towards their respective sides. The superior oblique draws the cornea down and out and rotates it inwardly. The inferior oblique draws the cornea up and rotates the eye outward. Any failure in the muscular system gives rise to double vision or other abnormality.

The four recti muscles surround the optic nerve between its exit from the skull and its entrance through the sclerotic coat behind the eyeball. The muscles themselves arise from the bony structure in the orbital region and are inserted into the appropriate portion of the sclerotic coat. The human eye lacks the retractor muscle present in almost all the lower mammals. As man has no third eyelid, a retractor muscle is less necessary.

THE OPTIC LENS

The lens, which lies immediately behind the iris, is suspended within its capsule from the *ciliary processes* by its suspensory ligament.

The ciliary processes are outshoots from the ciliary body, which is a ring of pigmented tissue lying around the inside of the eyeball joining up with and supporting the iris in front and connecting it with the choroid coat behind. It may be regarded as a direct continuation of the choroid coat, in an anterior direction. The lens is made up of many layers overlying each other like the coats of an onion. It is surrounded and held together by a homogenous, membranous capsule which is four or five times thicker in front than behind. The lens lies immediately behind the iris and its pupil, which contracts or dilates according to the amount of light falling on the retina.

The anterior surface of the human lens is slightly convex; the posterior surface is markedly so. This posterior portion fits into a corresponding cavity in the gelatinous, transparent substance contained in a thin, transparent capsule: the *hyaloid membrane*. The capsule and its jelly-like content forms what is known as the *vitreous body*. This forms about four-fifths of the total volume of the eye.

The capsule of the lens is attached to a circular muscle, the *ciliary muscle*, which is attached along its outer border to a ligament which unites it with the ciliary body. When the ciliary muscle contracts it tightens up the capsule of the lens and causes the lens to flatten somewhat; in other words to lose some of its convexity. This is the principle underlying what is known as *accommodation;* in other words focussing the lens to give a clear view of the object being examined. The ciliary muscle is more efficient in man than in most other animals.

THE IRIS

In man the pupil, the orifice through which light passes, is circular. In other animals it assumes various shapes which will be discussed later. The iris is pigmented, except in albinos, and is made up of circular fibres which close the pupil and radiating fibres, which open it. The central portion of the lens has the highest efficiency and the smaller the pupil is, at any moment, the sharper the visual image will be. This explains why a person who has poor accommodation and is greatly dependent upon glasses, is able to read small print by examining it through a pinhole made in a piece of black paper.

The colour of an iris may vary from black or dark brown to light blue. The deeper colouration is due to the presence of granules of the pigment melanin, but when pigment is absent the blood can be seen through the retaining layers of cells, and this gives rise to a blue colour.

INTRAOCULAR PRESSURE IN MAN AND OTHER ANIMALS

The canal of Schlemm, as represented in the lower animals, communicates with a second reticulate area, bounded by the pectinate ligament, the base of the iris and the cribriform ligament, all roofed

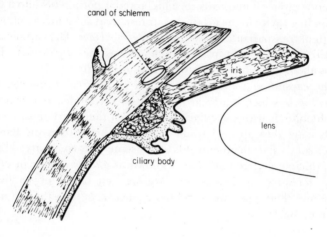

Fig. 13   The angle of the eye, and the canal of Schlemm.

in by the sclera. This cavity is made up of loose sponge-like tissue and in it are the Spaces of Fontana. This is present in horses, dogs and cats but is lacking in monkeys and man. The pectinate ligament is not well developed in any of the Primates but is porous and spongy and possesses numerous crypts leading into the stroma. In other animals it is dense and fibrous and does not play a direct part in fluid transmission. As a result, we find the epithelial covering of the ciliary processes exuding fluid into the anterior chamber and a complicated drainage system made up of the canal of Schlemm, the iris, the spaces of Fontana and the suprachoroidal space. When this mechanism remains normal and healthy, the intraorbital pressure remains at a fairly constant and satisfactory level.

If anything occurs which may interfere with the withdrawal of fluid, then the pressure within varies: it may rise (hypertony), or fall (hypotony). The flow of fluid into the venous plexus is in no way impeded by the action of the ciliary muscle owing to the fact that the outer portion of the cribriform ligament, being continuous with the sclera, acts as a buffer. Among the more common conditions which may interfere with the interchange of fluids are adhesions of the iris to the cornea or lens, displacement of the lens, conditions attending age with fibrosis and any condition affecting the cribriform ligament which may occlude the suprachoroidal space. Any softening of the vitreous humour may be another cause. The uveal tract is a term given to the vascular, pigmented membrane which forms the second layer of the eyeball. It includes the iris, choroid and ciliary body. These three structures have a very close affinity through continuity and contact but maintain a degree of independence on account of their various sources of blood supply. The uveal tract is the chief centre of nutrition of the eye and is therefore furnished with an excellent blood supply. It provides fluids which nourish the cornea and lens, and in the case of the horse, which lacks long retinal vessels, it assists in nourishing the retina also.

Thomson Henderson, one of the greatest ophthalmologists of the century, speaking in 1950 at the International Congress of the B.M.A. on the significance of pressure equilibrium on the intraocular contents, remarked that the level and nature of the intraocular pressure had been a fruitful source of discussion; on the other hand, the distribution of pressure in relation to the intraocular content had received scant attention. The balancing of intracranial pressure in relation to brain pressure had long been appreciated and the cerebrospinal fluid had been regarded as a single physiological unit, with the foramen of Magendi within the brain, as the connecting link between the lateral ventricles and the meninges, but no analogous provision had been made in the case of the eye.

The angle of the eye had been regarded as impervious to the passage of aqueous fluid into the suprachoroidal space. The retina and choroid were expected to transmit to the sclera a one-sided pressure, two and a half times that within the cranium, without any ill effects on the tissues of circulation. In the cranium on the other hand, such a unilateral pressure would give rise to pathological results by its effects upon tissues and circulation.

This led Thomson Henderson to believe that the angle was pervious to the passage of aqueous fluid into the suprachoroidal space and that pressure on the retina and choroid were not only blanced but were identical with that in the cranium so that, in man at least, no difference existed on either side of the lamina cribrosa.

In order to make the foregoing more easily understood, it may suffice to say that the cribriform ligament, being a sieve-like formation along the inner side of the canal of Schlemm, acts as a ligament of attachment to the ciliary muscle and is, therefore a constant feature, in contrast to the pectinate ligament, which exists only in the lower orders, in which the iris and ciliary base are compact, fibrous structures, terminating in front of the canal of Schlemm and requiring attachment. As mentioned earlier, in all mammals the cribriform ligament consists of a regular open network of longitudinal and circular fibres continuous with the inner lamellae of the cornea. Posterior to the canal of Schlemm the cribriform ligament divides into (a) outer fibres merging with those of the sclera, (b) inner fibres which are continued as the ciliary ligament. It is this bifurcation of the two portions of the cribriform ligament which forms the suprachoroidal space and provides the direct route by which aqueous fluid gains admission to it. In the human eye, in the absence of a functioning pectinate ligament, the iris terminates behind Schlemm's canal by direct attachment to the cribriform ligament. The so-called pectinate ligament of man and some of the other Primates, is in reality the cribriform ligament of the ciliary muscles, which follow the prescribed mammalian pattern and divide into scleral and muscular portions, providing direct passage to the suprachoroidal space. Man is the only animal in which the passage is not a direct one, owing to the presence behind Schlemm's canal, of the scleral ring.

THE RETINA

The retina can almost be accepted as being a portion of the brain which has extended through the optic nerve into the interior of the eye.

By means of the optic nerve the retina is connected to visual centres within the occipital lobe of the brain. From this, one may gather that images alighting on the surface of the retina, are conveyed along the tissues of the optic nerve to the appropriate part of the brain, and immediately translated into what we now term 'vision'. The site at the lower portion of the back of the retina through which the optic nerve makes its entry after passing through the sclera, is known as the optic disc. This is a grey or pinkish circular area about 5 mm in diameter in the human eye. In years gone by, it was known as the 'blind spot' because it was incapable of receiving any part of the visual image. Although we are not conscious of this blind area in our vision, it is present in every eye and there are ways in which its presence may be deomonstrated. A simple method is to hold a forefinger erect and about eighteen inches in front of the face. Close one eye and keep the other firmly fixed upon an object in front, such as a light bulb. Now keeping at the same distance from the face, move the finger and arm slowly to one side. You will find one position in which you can no longer see your finger, but on moving it a little farther, it will again appear. The point of disappearance corresponds with your blind spot.

The retina is the all-important part of the eye, for it is not only extremely light-sensitive but it is so wonderfully provided with nerve cells that it can pick up all the impressions which subscribe to the visual image and transmit these via the optic nerve to that portion of the brain which translates the impressions into the picture we finally visualise. Before the image upon the retina can be properly seen and appreciated, it is essential that the image should be focussed until the picture appears 'sharp'. In order to understand how this is effected, we must know something about the structure of the lens, which is rather peculiar.

The lens is a transparent structure and its purpose is to refract rays of light entering the eye, and bring them to a sharp focus on the retina, thus producing an image. The lens does not act alone in this respect but is assisted by some refraction from the curved cornea. In order to understand how the lens performs its functions we must first know something about its structure and its relationship to other parts of the eye.

When examined with the naked eye, the human lens appears as a smooth, transparent body, elastic in nature and about 1 cm in diameter and about 4 mm thick. Both its surfaces are convex, the posterior surface (facing the retina), more so than the anterior (facing the cornea). The two curved surfaces meet at the lens equator. The lens is surrounded by a tightly-fitting transparent, membranous capsule which is thicker over the anterior surface of the lens than over the posterior. The anterior surface of the vitreous is in contact with the posterior surface of the lens capsule, but without adhesion. However, when a cataract develops, the lens capsule and the vitreous may adhere which makes it difficult to remove the lens without taking with it some of the vitreous. However, when this occurs, the aqueous humour fills the gap.

Embryologically, the retina may be regarded as a part of the brain and optic nerve, which has extended over the inner surface of the choroid. It is by far the most sensitive and highly developed part of the whole eyeball. In its fresh state it is of a pale and translucent shade with the tapetum clearly visible beneath it.

The inner surface of the retina is opaque and is applied closely to the convexity of the hyaloid membrane which encloses the vitreous body, but it is in no way attached to this membrane. In the Primates the retina ceases anteriorly in a line termed the ora serrata but in the lower mammals it terminates in a continuous line which creates a smooth area between the retina and ciliary region which is termed the pars plana.

In all mammals the components of the ciliary region are arranged in an asymmetrical manner, the ciliary muscles, the pars plana and the ciliary processes are distributed unevenly. The asymmetry is on definite lines in each species of animal and is calculated to provide maximum efficiency by varying the latitude of vision in accordance with the needs of the animal's habits and environment. In quadrupeds the advantages gained by this disposition of the retina are amplified by the divergence existing in their optical axes. In the horse and many of the larger Herbivora in which the large foreface occludes downward vision (even when the head is held normally), the superior field of vision is always the greater. This is advantageous when the animal is grazing. When a ruminant is using its horns in combat and the horns are very upright or directed backward, as in some deer, vision must be practically occluded. This is why some varieties in combat interlock their horns rather than charging down upon each other. In Carnivora, in which the degree of optical divergence is less, the retina does not come far forward so that the temporal quadrant is more extensive than the nasal quadrant.

The fibres of the optic nerve run from the retinal ganglion cells and converge upon the optic disc which is the point at which they leave the eye. The 'blind spot' in the human eye arises owing to the fact that the nerve fibres at this point pass back through the retina, thus creating a small area in which both rods and cones are absent. The blind spot is never centrally placed. In most domesticated animals it lies a little nearer the temporal side of the retina but in

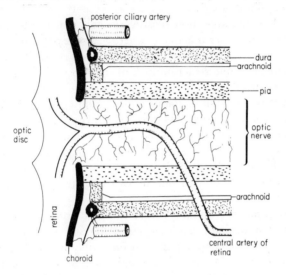

Fig. 14 Schematic representation of course of central artery into optic nerve.

the Primates it lies nearer the nasal canthus. Through the ophthalmoscope it appears as a disc-like elevation in the form of a thick ring, ranging from white to salmon pink in colour. From the centre of the periphery comparatively large blood vessels emerge and radiate over the surface of the retina. The number of vessels and their disposition on the retina, together with whether they emerge from the centre of the disc or from its edges and the distance they travel, enables the trained observer to determine which animal type is under observation.

The central fovea is a small depression shaped like a shallow bowl with a concave floor, on the vitreal face of the retina. It is derived from a bending of the layers 5–9 of the retina and a thickening of the bacillary and outer nuclear layers. From edge to edge in the human eye it is $1500\,\mu$ across while its central floor measures $400\,\mu$

across. The central part of the fovea consists wholly of cones, longer and thinner than anywhere else in the retina, The macula, usually referred to as the *yellow spot* or macula lutea, is an ill-defined area of the central retina containing a yellow pigment in the nerve layers. It extends over the whole of the central portion of the retina, but the intensely pigmented part is confined to the fovea.

In man and monkeys the most sensitive part of the retina is the macula. It is the area most sensitive to light but in darkness or a dim light, it becomes practically useless. Actually the fovea in man is comparatively elementary. It is shallow and concave when compared with the same structure in birds and lizards. Its magnifying effect is practically nil. The fovea centralis is the centre of the human macula. It is yellowish in colour and certainly during the hours of daylight is quite effective. The fovea is not constantly present in all vertebrates. It is common in the bony fishes and in a large number of the teleostei (trout, herring, perch, goldfish) but is most evident and well developed in lizards. It is absent in frogs, crocodiles and most of the turtle family. With one or two exceptions, it is absent in snakes.

Histologically the retina is a very complex structure and is made up from ten distinguishable layers. Although it is transparent, photochemically changing pigments in purple, red and orange, all of which absorb light, are distinguishable and these are the primary agents in developing the processes which give rise to the phenomenon we term 'sight'. The most important part of the retina is that situated adjacent to the choroidal surface. The area which first receives the light rays is composed of nervous tissue derived from the optic nerve. The light travels through almost the entire thickness of the retina before reaching the rods and cones, which are away from the light. The pigmented epithelium is farthest from the source of light. This is referred to as an inverted structure and it exists in all vertebrate retinae.

Chemical changes take place in the cells of the retina as the result of changes in light intensity but it is not certain whether these changes favour light reception and the excitation of nervous impulses. The retina may also be stimulated by electrical changes but the significance of such activity is not yet fully understood.

The retina makes its responses to light changes but all other stimulii produce the same general type of light response, in darkness as well as in light.

CONSTRUCTION OF THE RETINA

The layers of the retina, commencing from the outer (choroidal) surface, are:

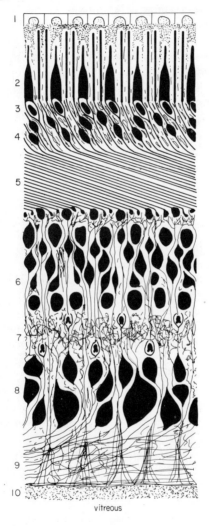

vitreous

Fig. 15   Section of a human eye (numbers of sections correspond
with numbers in text).

(1) Burk's membrane
(2) Pigmented epithelium. A layer of polygonal pigmented cells, usually six-sided. These are unpigmented in the area occupied by the tapetum fibrosum.
(3) Receptor outer segment
(4) Receptor inner segment
In the above two layers, the rods, being longer, extend vertically between the first and third layers; the cones, being much shorter, do not extend downwards as far as the pigmented epithelium.
(5) Membrana limitans externa. This forms the boundary of the framework of fibres supporting.
(6) The outer nuclear layer
(7) The outer plexiform layer
(8) The inner nuclear layer
(9) The inner plexiform layer
(10) Ganglion cell layer
(11) Nerve fibre layer.

These are the fibres of the optic nerve which have passed through the lamina cribrosa (so far as it exists in the lower animals), and having lost their medullary sheaths, at the point of entrance into the eyeball, are now radiating over the internal surface. They are supported by:
(12) Membrana limitans interna.
This is the inner boundary of the sustenacular framework which supports the nervous elements in the preceding layers. Altogether, six types of neurones go to make up the nervous structure of the retina (a) rod and cone visual cells (b) neurones of the first order, (c) bipolar cells, neurones of the second order (d) Ganglion cells (e) neurones the third order and (f) horizontally arranged neurones.

RODS AND CONES

Rods and cones are the names given to the nerve cells in the retina which react to light. They are of two kinds, narrow cylindrical rods and the shorter, stouter cones. Many thousands of these are packed on top of the pigmented epithelium which forms the deepest layer of the retina, sometimes mixed and in other parts in distinct groups. Generally speaking, the rods are adapted to night vision and the

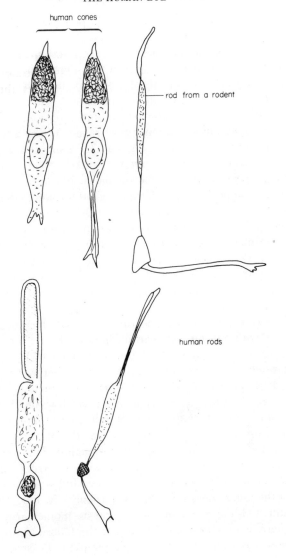

human cones

rod from a rodent

human rods

Fig. 16   Rods and cones.

cones to daylight and colour vision. Rods are more numerous in the
central area of high visual activity. Both rods and cones come into
action in daylight; the cones, centrally situated, being employed to

examine for detail, and the rods at the periphery, being employed to size up moving objects.

Human beings find it easier to discern a distant light or a small star if they do not look straight at it but slightly to one side or the other, in order to divert the light away from the rods (which probably would not register it), to the cones.

Travelling a little lower down the evolutionary scale, let us imagine a cat staring at a mouse at fairly close range, in such a way that the light rays impinge upon a point of the retina close to the optic disc. The eyes of a cat are not particularly good at short range vision and we will presume that the mouse has started to run away. Its image now begins to pass from the central cones to the peripheral rods, so the cat can see it better. Similarly, a man walking down a street may notice a lot of other folk in a casual way since he is using peripheral vision and rods do not register an impression very definitely. Perhaps another person staring at him from the pavement hails him. He turns his head slightly in response and fixes the image of his acquaintance onto the central portion of the retina, making full use of the rods.

The cat is by nature a nocturnal animal. Her eyes are well provided with rods but her central cones are scanty. A terrier would not lose sight of a mouse at a range of four feet in daylight but a cat would catch mice at night that the terrier would never see. Both dogs and cats as well as a good many human beings, may fail to see a stationary object of comparatively small size, unless they bump into it. Perhaps this is not quite so true of the cat as it is of the dog, for several reasons. One is that the dog places the sense of smell before that of sight and will sometimes fall over the game it is retrieving before it actually recognises it. A cat will flick the live mouse it is carrying away several feet and wait for it to move. When the mouse does this, the cat recognises it. But, if the mouse lies still and the attention of the cat is momentarily attracted elsewhere, it may be unable to locate the mouse again. Thinking the prey has escaped, the cat will jump to the spot where she expects the mouse to be. The interval may have given the mouse a welcome opportunity to escape.

Many hypermetropic humans, people with what is termed 'long sight', see rather badly by day when they are depending on their cones but see quite normally by night within the normal limitations imposed by near darkness. Night vision is also bound up with chemical changes in the rods, which are essential. Rhodopsin or Visual purple, is an unstable reddish pigment which is developed in the outer segment of the rods during darkness. It is believed that only the rods are concerned in this process but a second pigment, Visual violet, has been recorded in the cones. (Thomson Henderson). It is believed that this latter pigment is not of great importance in night vision. During daylight the eye becomes light adapted and an eye protected from light becomes dark adapted.

CHAPTER 4

THE EYE OF THE DOG

There are few animals which exhibit such a variety of eye shapes as the dog family. One encounters the large, protruding, badly protected eye of the Pekinese; the 'varminty' eyes of the Terriers, with very little eye protruding through the lids. There are various intermediate stages laid down for particular breeds, nearly three hundred of them. One must remember that the domestic dog has become an artificial representative of its early progenitors and that all breeds from minute Chihuahua to the St Bernard have all been created by preserving and interbreeding all the freak mutations which have appeared through the centuries.

As compared with the eye of man, that of the dog is somewhat smaller, although the lens of the canine eye is relatively very much larger, which makes lens extraction in the dog a more difficult procedure. In man the proportion in the size of lens and eyeball is 1:18. In the dog it is 1:10·2.

THE PALPEBRAL FISSURE

This term refers to the space between the eyelids when the eye is fully open. Its shape and relationship varies greatly in different breeds. Congenital narrowness is admired in Terriers with very little of the cornea visible. In Pekinese, the eye is round and it bulges to such an extent that it frequently ulcerates through over exposure to wind, rain and frost, apart from dust and foreign bodies. When the palpebral fissure is too wide, as in Bloodhounds and St Bernards, the lower eyelid may droop giving rise to ectropion. In Chows and several other breeds, a superfluity of skin around the eyes gives rise to turning-in of the eyelids which causes the eyelashes to impinge on the cornea and set up intense irritation. This condition is known as entropion. The breed standards issued by breed clubs for the information of their members lays down the nature of the abnormality required in the particular breed, irrespective as to whether it harbours good for the dog or ill.

Each eyelid is built up of a framework of dense connective tissue, the tarsal plate. On its outer surface the plate is covered by skin and lined on its inner surface by conjunctiva. The lids are moulded to the shape of the eyeball. Opening and closing the palpebral fissure is carried out mainly by movements of the upper eyelid. The lower is inactive until the upper lid closes when it may tighten up and firmly close the fissure by contraction of the orbicularis muscle which surrounds the eyelids. In birds the lower eyelid does all the work. In the dog the lashes grow from the external half of the upper lid and normally there are none in the lower lid. When hairs do grow here they often cause irritation of the eyeball. Immediately behind the eyelashes of the upper lid is a row of black dots, the openings of the *Meibomian* glands which secrete sebaceous material which lubricates the edges of the lids. There are about 40 of these openings in the dog.

THE CORNEA

The anterior, transparent coat of the eyeball, continuous with the sclerotic is exposed to more stress in many breeds of dog than in man because it either protrudes with insufficient lid coverage, or it is almost hidden behind lids, without free drainage. It suffers, especially in the shortfaced breeds, from inflammation (keratitis) and from ulceration. In Pekinese a little rough handling or traction upon the 'scruff' of the neck may cause prolapse of the eyeball. This is due to the amount of proptosis present—the amount of corneal (and sometimes sclerotic) surface exposed to the weather.

While in the majority of animals the cornea is slightly elliptical and rather wider in the transverse direction, that of the dog is roughly circular with seldom more than 1 mm increase in the transverse direction.

THE LENS

In the dog the lens is relatively larger than in man and is almost equally convex at front and back.

In man the lens is flatter in front and more markedly curved at the rear.

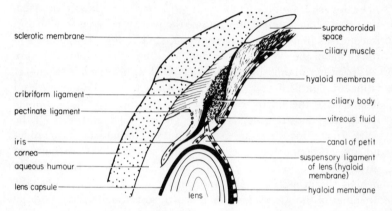

Fig. 17   Lens suspension in the dog. The hyaloid membrane which encloses the vitreous humour, travels over the ciliary processes and divides into two parts just above the lens periphery. This is continued over the lens capsule to form the suspensory ligament of the lens. Another name for the suspensory ligament is the Zonule of Zinn.

THE RETINA

In man and the anthropoid apes there exists a pigmented area in the retina known as the *macula lutea* near the centre of which lies a depression, the *fovea centralis*. This corresponds with the spot at which the rays of light passing through the centre of the pupil, fall upon the retina. The macula lutea is composed almost wholly of cones and is regarded as the most acute visual area of the retina. In the dog, and in other mammals the fovea is absent but hypersensitive areas can be mapped out in some of these, although they cannot be detected when the retina is examined through an ophthalmoscope. In the dog and cat the hypersensitive area is a rounded or horizontally elliptical area immediately external to the optic disc. This can be seen through the ophthalmoscope as a glistening golden-yellow area, free from large blood vessels, lying below the transverse vessels on

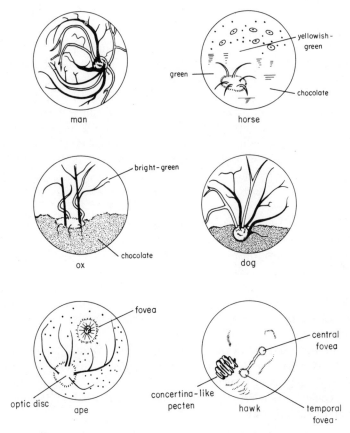

Fig. 17(a) Fundus of the eye in several animals. In the ape the
fovea is visible, as is the optic disc. In the hawk there are two
foveae, one central, the other temporal. A concertina-like pecten
is also present.

the temporal side of the retina, that is, the side nearer the cheek
of the dog. Unfortunately the dog has no colour vision. In the dog,
in company with most of the Carnivora, beneath the retina and
superimposed upon the choroid coat, there lies a layer of iridescent
shining cells, known as iridocytes. All but two species of Carnivora
and the Seal family possess this type of tapetum, known as the
tapetum cellulosum.

Viewed through the ophthalmoscope, the tapetum of a dog exhibits
a bronze, metallic lustre, tapering away to blue or white at its edges,

but the variations in old animals, young animals, and in different breeds, may be marked. It is believed that the tapetum, which reflects back the light passing through the pupil, may assist vision by re-transmitting the image on to the back of the retina. In the dog the tapetum may occupy a large or quite a small portion of the fundus (a term relating to the depths of the eyeball). It may even assume a ribbon-like shape. It may or may not include the optic disc.

The lower portion of the tapetum, (the tapetum nigrum), in the dog is usually darker in colour and in Pekinese and Pugs the tapetum may contain granules of melanin giving it a chocolate coloured appearance, sometimes interspersed with black. In eyes affected with progressive retinal atrophy this dark staining may arise from damage to the blood vessels which traverse the retina.

In a healthy eye these vessels, arteries and veins, penetrate the wall of the eye through the optic disc and spread over the surface of the retina in the form of three or four main trunks giving off branches. See Fig. 17(a). In progressive retinal atrophy, these vessels gradually disappear and the retina is then supplied with blood only by subsidiary vessels. The result is permanent blindness. Progressive retinal atrophy is regarded as a hereditary disease in dogs. (See later chapter.)

The rods and cones present in the human retina, for example, have different functions. They represent the visual cells. The rods, being longer, extend vertically between the first and third layers. The cones are much shorter cells, and they do not extend downwards as far as the tapetum.

THE IRIS

In the dog the iris is remarkable in that it fails to contract its pupil when small objects are viewed at close range, as happens in most other mammals, but it dilates instead. The aperture, apart from size remains the same shape during contraction, that is to say the pupil is circular. The iris is striated and carries circular markings which correspond with the contraction of constrictor muscle fibres of concentric pattern, especially when the pupil of the eye changes its diameter. In this way the iris of the dog (and some other mammals) carries a distinctive pattern which may be typed and classified as finger prints are. Attempts have been made in U.S.A. and some other countries to use these facts as a method of identification.

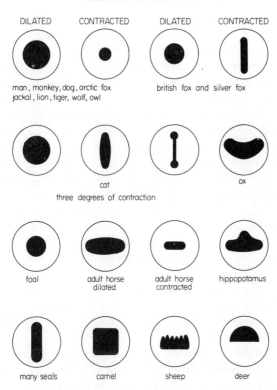

Fig. 18 Pupil shape in various animals.

In the foxes related to the dog family, the iris behaves differently in different species. In the common wild fox, of this country, the pupil contracts to an upright narrow slit. It does this too in the Silver Fox. But in the Fennec—the nocturnal fox of North Africa, the pupil is large and round, and the same applies to the Arctic Fox, which has pupils resembling those of the domestic dog. The Jackal, one of the animals from which the dog may have descended also has round pupils.

ACCOMMODATION IN MAMMALS

With the exception of the horse, in particular, and some of the ungulates, the theory generally accepted as regards the method adopted in order to focus the eyes, is as follows:

The ciliary muscle contracts and by so doing the anterior part of the choroid layer is drawn forward, bringing the apices of the ciliary processes closer together. In this way the tension of the suspensory ligament of the lens slackens and the elastic lens, which has hitherto been compressed, begins to bulge, chiefly at its anterior surface which is the part more firmly held under compression by the suspensory layer (Zonule of Zinn). The anterior surface of the lens is also free from the compression exercised upon it by the vitreous body, on which the hinder part of the lens is moulded. The whole action is put into reverse by relaxation of the ciliary muscle. The ciliary muscle is unevenly distributed around the ciliary circumference, and this fact has been regarded as conducive to astigmatism.

In most animals the iris plays a part in securing accommodation. Usually it contracts while the eye is focusing and relaxes when the eye is at rest. The dog is exceptional in this respect as it reverses the process, allowing the pupil to dilate when viewing objects at close range.

Many of the smaller monkeys make use of what is termed 'the stenopaic pupil', that is to say they reduce the aperture of the pupil almost to pinpoint size and examine objects held in the hands, for instance, at a range of a few inches giving the impression that they are short-sighted (myopic) when they are actually hypermetropic or long-sighted. Although the dog fails in this respect, the cat (like the camel) is able to close its pupil to pin-point diameter.

The method of accommodation practised by humans and rather less accurately by some of the lower mammals, varies considerably among other animals such as the birds and the fishes and will be discussed in connection with each species.

In man, dogs, cats, and many other mammals, the light rays entering the eye through the pupil meet precisely on the retina. Vision is then good. This is termed *emmetropia*.

If the rays meet in front of the retina, the vision is blurred and a condition of short sight (or *myopia*) occurs. If the rays meet behind the retina, a condition of long sight (hypermetropia) exists.

Smith (1921) wrote 'All objects having the same visual angle form the same-sized picture on the retina. By the aid of the visual angle the size of the image on the retina may be calculated, provided we know the distance of the nodal point (the centre of curvature of the refracting surface) from the retina; thus, at the distance of a mile, a man six feet in height, is represented on the retina of a horse by an image 1/880th of an inch in height. In a human eye at the same distance, the picture of a man would be 1/1500th of an inch, or about the size of a red corpuscle.' The nearer the object,

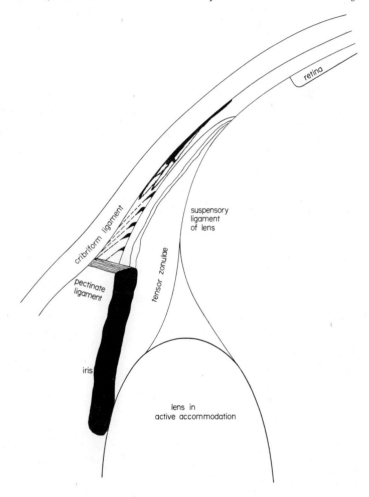

Fig. 19 Section of part of the eye of a wolf in active accommodation.

the larger will be the image. If a six foot man were viewed by a dog at a distance of 110 yards, the image on the dog's retina would be about one eighth of an inch. It may be presumed that a moderate

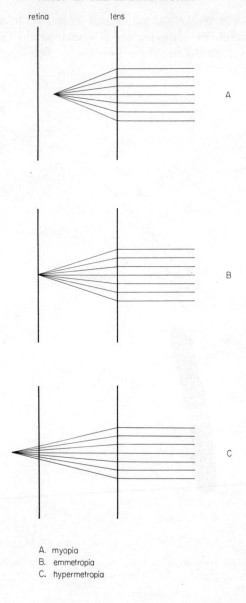

A. myopia
B. emmetropia
C. hypermetropia

Fig. 20 Defects in vision.

degree of hypermetropia exists normally in wild mammals, particularly in those which catch their prey.

A good deal of discussion has waged throughout the years regarding how well or how badly a dog makes use of its ciliary muscle in the act of accommodation and the general belief is that the ability of a dog to focus does not compare favourably with that

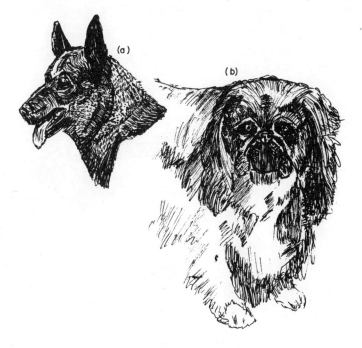

Fig. 21 Monocular and binocular vision in the same species:
In (a) the vision is lateral, the eyes being approximately 30°
with the median line of the head.
In (b) the vision is frontal, the eyes being approximately 90°
with the line of the head.

in man. But the fact remains that a greyhound sees a moving rabbit a hundred and fifty yards ahead although it may not recognise one lying motionless in a grass field at twenty yards distance. Against this one must remember that a dog is colour blind and the shade of grey in which it would see a rabbit may tone in very closely with that of the surrounding foliage so that the contrast we would see would be denied the dog.

On the other hand, although many dogs fail to observe objects
upon the ground, gundogs trained in bird work, will recognise
moving birds at great heights in spite of the fact that birds in the air
are not approaching or leaving fixed objects as animals are when
moving through a field. Then again when looking upwards a terrier
will develop the ability to catch particles of meat or biscuit tossed to
it from several yards away with seldom a failure. Coming from all

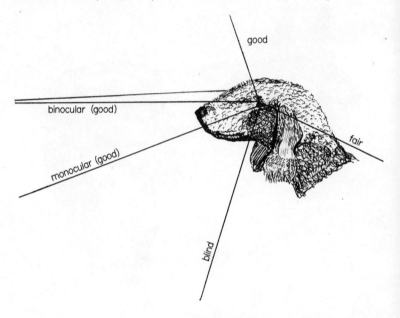

Fig. 22   Bedlington Terrier: in the dog family, visual acuity
varies with the breed.

directions the quality of vision to enable a dog to see such small
objects in flight and judge the spot at which they will land, must
be very high. Moving objects are not visualised so much on the
centre of the retina as upon its periphery. It may well be that a
dog depends upon vision for more distant objects but prefers to use
its delicate sense of smell to locate near objects rather than depend
upon vision.

It is, however, practically hopeless to endeavour to direct a dog's
vision by means of the pointing finger, even when one points
upwards. The dog will concentrate on the outstretched hand, or
ignore it, but in either case it seldom gets the message. Nor does

it look in a mirror placed at eye level or take an interest in the television screen. It may be attracted by another dog barking but does not see that dog. This is based on my own experience after testing large numbers of dogs, although when I drew attention to this in a daily paper I received over a hundred letters from readers whose dogs, they stated, took a great interest in television and would walk up to the screen when dogs and cats were on view and attempt to touch them. This merely proves that there are at least a hundred dogs in Great Britain which are attracted by the television screen, but millions which are not.

Greyhounds which catch and kill are usually hypermetropic in some degree. In individual dogs tested by me from $0.5D$[1] to $1.5D$ was common, but in rare cases the degree of hypermetropia in a racing dog might be $3.5D$. Contrary to general opinion, myopia in Greyhounds appears to be rare.

From $0.75D$ to $1.5D$ does not interfere with viewing a *moving* rabbit or hare and the range of distant vision in the Greyhound is incomparable and far superior to that in any of the other gazehounds. Some of the brachycephalic, (the short-headed, flat faced breeds), notably the Pekinese which have large, prominent eyes, fail to recognise their owners at a distance of 25 feet.

Dogs vary very greatly according to their breed as to whether they see objects with one eye at a time (monocular vision) or with two eyes (binocular vision). Only a few breeds, including some of the Toys, the Pekinese, Maltese and Pug as examples, have frontally placed eyes and binocular vision. The majority of breeds have eyes set on either side of a high forehead with a tendency to look sideways rather than directly forwards. Some of the Gazehounds, with narrow foreheads more nearly approach frontality as do some of the Terriers, but the majority of the larger breeds possess binocular vision. This is made easier in many cases by the possession of a long, supple neck which can alter the position of the head to enable it to use its eyes alternately to the best advantage.

If we place a dog on a table and persuade it to look straight ahead and we then draw an imaginary line through the plane of the right eye and another through the plane of the left eye, we can imagine these lines meeting behind the dog's head. The angle at which these lines meet will be the dog's 'visual angle'. The visual angles

---

[1] D = Diopter; a diopter is the unit of power of a lens. A convergent lens of 1 metre focal length is said to have a power of $+1$ Diopter.

in Terriers is usually from 18–25 degrees as compared with 5–10 degrees in Pekinese. In the cat the angle is 8–18 degrees. In Man it is nil. In order to possess good stereoscopic vision, binocular vision is indispensable.

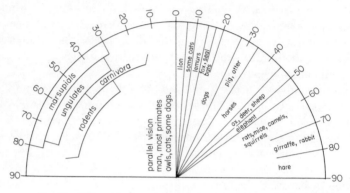

Fig. 23   The approximate angles of vision in certain animals
(After Thomson Henderson).

VISION IN THE DOG

There are approximately 300 breeds of dogs, all different. Eye placement varies from that in which vision can only be monocular, to that in the brachycephalic types which have nearly frontal vision.

It is difficult to decide whether those with frontal vision see as well, less well, or better, than those which see only with one eye most of the time, since the dogs with frontal vision are nearly all pets, more or less housebound and seldom called upon even to see across the road alone. The general impression is that these dogs have very inferior vision for distance but it must be remembered that most of them are very close to the ground. During most of their walks on a lead the world must appear as a forest of legs.

Most of the gazehounds rely mainly upon monocular vision, but they have the advantage of a long flexible neck which enables them to switch almost instantaneously from eye to eye. However, their vision for distant objects which are still is not outstanding, but they have good vision for a moving object which they keep in view as long as the movement continues. Dogs seem to have better vision for objects above eye level. They will watch a snipe or a bird flying overhead and can recognise a tall owner at a considerable distance. On the whole the Terrier family appear to possess the best all-round vision.

Although a great many of the Toy breeds, such as the Chihuahua and the Pekinese, often spending much of their time in the arms of their owner, may appear to possess somewhat imperfect vision and to be rather short-sighted, this may be due in part to the fact that they have no particular need to depend upon their eyes and are quite content to rely upon their sense of smell when investigating objects close at hand.

But it would appear that dogs, like children, can be educated and taught to notice objects they would not trouble about if they were left entirely to their own devices. If dogs are talked to in the way that one talks to young children, and persuaded to take notice of objects to which their attention is repeatedly drawn, they develop in a very short time a great improvement in their power of convergence and perhaps show a similar rise in their intelligence quotient.

Puppies do not usually open their eyes until about the tenth day after birth. During this interval the eye is completing its final stages of development, something which in the human eye is done before the date of birth. Another change at this time involves the blood vessels of the embryonic eye in which a blood vessel—the hyaloid artery—which has entered the eyeball at the optic papilla, spreads a network of arterioles throughout the vitreous body (which it nourishes), spread over the posterior surface of the optic lens. After this vessel has become absorbed, a canal is left in the vitreous humour, quite narrow in the dog's eye but maintaining a permanent diameter of 2–3 mm in the horse. Sometimes the absorption is not quite complete and some fine filaments may remain in the vitreous of the adult eye.

It is due to this similar phenomenon that some people complain of 'floaters' when they stare into space, especially upon a clear and sunny day. Normal folk ignore these floaters but psychopaths and some introspective humans regard them as a serious handicap. Occasionally one sees a dog—but more frequently a cat—which has a habit of sitting in the sunshine apparently 'catching flies', with its fore feet. It is possible such animals are seeing 'floaters', relics of an incompletely absorbed hyaloid artery—free in the substance of the vitreous body.

Usually two or three weeks may elapse after the eyes open before the puppy is able to recognise the other members of the litter, or the person who looks after it. Usually the first object it recognises and understands is its food dish. At about the fourth week, it begins to recognise its litter mates and shows signs of associating with them and indulging in play. It has by then learned not to walk into solid obstacles but it still has little recognition of what visual images represent and their true form or solidity.

Definition of the retina in the dog occurs much later in the stage of development than it does in man. The retinae of new-born pups are essentially non-vascular and blood vessels first make their appearance about seventeen days after birth or about one week after the eyes open. Parry (1953) observed no striking difference in the retinae of dogs which hunted by sight or by sense of smell, but in each he recognised the likelihood of an area in the retina which possessed only cones.

In the dog the retina is believed to derive its nourishment primarily from the vascular layer of the choroid but as in all mammals, the vessels passing out from the optic papilla and radiating over the inner surface of the retina play a part. These nourish the internal layers of the retina which consist of a single layer of multi-polar nerve cells and a layer of nerve fibres of the optic nerve which have lost their medullary sheaths at the point of entrance to the eyeball and are now radiating over the internal surface of the retina supported by its internal membrane.

The reason that so much attention has been devoted to the nourishment of the retina is because numbers of dogs bred for exhibition are now developing Progressive Retinal Atrophy, with disappearance of the vessels radiating over the internal surface of the retina and a progressive loss of vision. This is regarded as a hereditary disease.

CHAPTER 5

THE EYE OF THE CAT

The cat possesses an open orbit, differing slightly from that of the dog as it is more constricted in its middle portion where the orbital ligament divides it into two parts, one containing the eyeball, and

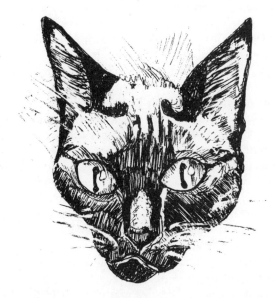

Fig. 24   The eyes of the cat showing the stenopaic pupil consisting of a narrow vertical slit with a pinhole aperture at each extremity.

the hinder part the upper end of the lower jawbone. The palpebral orifice, the space between the eyelids, is larger and more circular in the cat than in any but the short-faced varieties of dog, and the whole of the cornea is exposed when the eye is fully open.

One of the other differences between the eye of dog and cat is that the pupil in the cat's eye is completely circular when dilated in a dim light but, unlike that of the dog, it does not retain its circular outline when contracted, but contracts to a narrow, upright slit with a minute circular opening at either end of the slit: the so-called stenopaic apertures. Not only does the pupil dilate in a dim light, but whenever the cat becomes angry, excited, or even when it is frightened, a slit pupil makes its appearance in the form of an erect oval, usually without sufficient contraction to exhibit the terminal apertures. (See Fig. 18.)

The third eyelid in the cat is a thin, pink or whitish, neatly fitting structure, which may remain slightly visible even when the eye is widely opened. In a cat which is unwell or in one which has been starved, the membrana nictitans may be wholly or partly drawn over the eye, permanently. This is due to loss of fat at the back of the eyeball which causes the eye to retract, thus causing the third eyelid to rise and cover the cornea. The tapetum in the cat is yellow to green in colour and its reflection can be seen from a considerable distance at night when a torch or the lights of a car shine through the pupils.

The vascularity of the tapetum itself is practically nil except for the small capillaries which traverse vertically and show through the ophthalmoscope as minute dark, sometimes bright and sometimes concentric rings, to which the name of Stars of Wimslow, has been given. The Siamese cat may possess a chocolate coloured tapetum, or it may be absent and instead of a tapetum one may observe a pink colouration arising from the capillaries in the choroid under-lying the retina, reminiscent of the 'camp fire' glow from the human eye. The papilla—the optic disc—in the cat is circular, salmon-pink in colour and surounded by an indigo ring. The arteries and veins crossing the retina, radiate from the periphery of the disc, instead of from its centre as in the dog.

The optical divergence of an eye is a measure of the degree of lateral vision associated with the position of the eyes in the head.

Man is said to have parallel vision with no optical divergence, owing to the situation of his eyes. The cat, however, has an optical divergence of only 5–10 degrees which is as near frontality as one is likely to find except in the Primates.

The big cats, the lions and tigers, kept in cages in zoological collections, very quickly develop abnormal vision owing to a gradual atrophy of the ciliary muscles and would be unable, if liberated to make normal use of their eyes, in the manner that they would be able to if the extent of their vision was full. This does not apply to animals kept in National Parks or other establishments with free range. These larger cats all have round pupils, whether dilated or contracted. Animals which have the advantage of numerous rods in

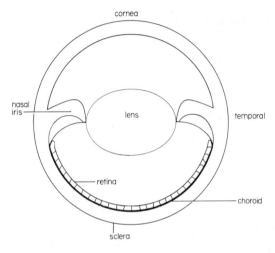

Fig. 25   The eye of a cat (horizontal section). Note that it is not symmetrical: the temporal side is considerably larger than the nasal and probably extends the peripheral zone of vision. In this illustration the pupil is fully dilated as when hunting by night.

their retinae have the best possible nocturnal vision for prowling and hunting during the hours of darkness.

Diurnal animals will possess an abundance of cones. In the human retina there are about twenty times as many cones as rods. The macula in the human eye contains nothing but cones and is of the greatest value when one wants to examine an object in close detail. While the cones are used in this way, the rods may be employed in daylight to catch a glimpse of objects 'out of the corner' of the eye. Cats are provided both with cones and rods, though the number of cones is limited.

A cat may fail to see a mouse motionless, against a grey background, but when the mouse runs its image may be visible as it crosses the cat's cones and the cat may then catch it and play with it. If the mouse should escape to a distance of three to four feet it may take cover, or remain free until it again moves. Apparently the cat's vision is at its best between six and eighteen feet in front of its eyes. Nocturnal vision is always short range vision and no eyes, however good, can penetrate complete darkness. Cats usually move at a leisurely pace and make their spring when they find themselves within striking distance. They prefer to lie in wait rather than hunt like a dog or a fox.

It is apparent that in both dogs and cats the ability to judge distance (how far away, for example, a moving car is at any given moment) is sometimes learned only by experience and even then cats and dogs seldom realise that mechanical vehicles move much more rapidly than they themselves can. It is doubtful whether animals have the ability to recognise or evaluate perspective and use it as a guide to determining whether objects are near or distant. Nor, probably, have they our ability to recognise that objects nearer the horizon begin to fade or take on a lighter hue. It is unlikely their eyes ever look very far ahead or that horizons hold any great interest for them. The cat has better long distance vision by day than even the brachycephalic dogs, which have almost frontal vision and can recognise objects thirty yards distant.

The remarkable feature is that an animal so nearly nocturnal should also enjoy such good vision by day. It is helped both by night and day by the extreme mobility of its pupil which can vary from an elongated vertical slit to a round aperture as large as the cornea itself. It seems likely that when the pupil is fully contracted the cat may be able to see without any attempt at accommodation, much after the style of the pin-hole camera which requires no adjustment so long as the light is good, or the instamatic type of camera which has a short focal length. In any case the ciliary muscle in the eye of the cat is rather elementary when compared with that in the human eye and it is likely that better definition can be provided by regulating the size of the pupil than by adjusting the curvature of the lens.

Davson in his *Physiology of the Eye*, states that colour vision in the cat has been well studied, perhaps because of its status as a domestic pet, and certainly because of the use of its ganglion cells for study of unit activity. Behaviourly, Daw and Periman (1970) have been able to establish discrimination between red and cyan, and orange and cyan; this was at liminance levels and saturated the rods so that one must postulate two types of cone at least. Some lateral geniculate units were found showing opponent properties suggesting inputs from green and blue-absorbing photoreceptors, so that evidence suggests that the cat is a dichromat and more specifically, a tritanonalous protanope. The dichromat is one who can match all colours with suitable mixtures of only two, instead of three primaries. A protanope is one who is missing the fundamental red sensation: he is red blind.

CHAPTER 6

THE EYE OF
THE HORSE

VISION IN THE HORSE

So far we have discussed only the open orbit as it exists in the dog and cat. The depth and shape of the orbit varies in the different species of animals and the degree of protection afforded by the bony casing. This is greater in man, in the higher apes and in most of the herbivorous animals but is incomplete in the pig, in which it resembles that of the dog. The orbit in the horse is closed.

In the horse, the internal wall of the orbit and the anterior third of its floor, are made up from the cranial bones and those of the face; while the superior and outer parts of the orbit comprise only the orbital arch which is a ring of bone made up out of the supraorbital process of the frontal bone, which replaces the orbital ligament of the dog, and the zygoma, or that part of it derived from the malar bone. The eye occupies the portion of the orbital cavity anterior to the supraorbital process while the coronoid process, the upper end of the ramus of the lower jawbone, occupies that portion of the orbital cavity posterior to the supraorbital process.

It is rather curious that in the ungulates, only those which fight with horns, make use of the superior strength of the closed orbit. One can only suppose that a creature which had to contend with kicks, and blows such as might be contracted by an animal compelled to make an escape by galloping, might receive violent blows on the head which made the closed orbit necessary. When a horse does meet with an orbital injury with risk of infection, it is not uncommonly a cause of death. It might well be that during the evolutionary development of the horse, those with the stronger and best protected orbits survived and reproduced their kind, while those with less complete protection were wiped out.

80

It must be realised that an open or closed orbit is not necessarily related to eye position, for we find cats with eyes frontally placed and rabbits and hares with open orbits, but generally speaking, open orbits are associated with animals that have a wide gape, although rabbits and hares hardly come under this category. The dog with frontal eye placement between 5 and 35 degrees has the open orbit, but the horse which has similar eyes as regards optical divergence, has entirely different orbits.

THE EYEBALL

In the horse the eyeball is asymmetrical, the cornea being situated a little nearer the upper than the lower part of the eye. The horse possesses a ramp retina. This means that the retinal surface is tilted

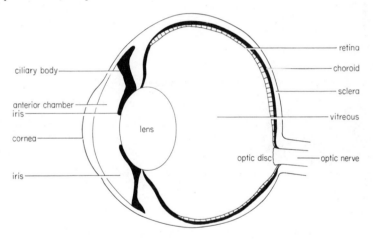

Fig. 26   Vertical section of the left eye of the horse, with dilated pupil.

relative to the visual axis of the eye. This is equivalent to sloping the plate in a camera so that objects at varying distances from the plate can all be brought into sharp focus, as when one photographs a tall building from ground level, thus, the retina slopes so that its upper part is farther from the lens than the lower part. The ciliary muscle in the horse plays only a very small part in varying the degree of lens convexity.

Accommodation at varying distances is achieved almost wholly by head movements which direct the visual image onto the most suitable part of the ramp retina, according to whether the eye is viewing a near or distant object. By this means, a sharp retinal image can be obtained without altering the shape of the lens. It must be realised, however, that a horse ridden at, and over jumps can focus accurately only when it is given free head movement.

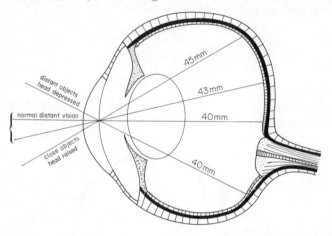

Fig. 27   Section of the eye of the horse showing how it contrives to focus upon objects simply by raising or lowering the head, in order that light impinges on a different portion of the retina. The surface of the retina does not form a true arc of the circle. It is 'ramped' so that the view becomes clear when the head is raised into an appropriate position and the rays of light fall upon the most suitable part of the retinal surface. The retina thus provides a different focal length with every change in the position of the head. A horse approaching a jump can only be certain of its position and height, if given free movement of the head.

The cornea of the horse, is 35 mm wide and measures only 28·5 mm in the vertical direction. The globe of the eye measures 34 mm across and 50·5 mm from above to below. The surface of the cornea to the retina is approximately 44 mm, but as we are dealing with a ramp retina, this measurement will vary very slightly; that from the centre of the cornea to the upper part of the retina being 45 mm, and from the centre of the cornea to the centre of the retina, only 43 mm. The distance from the centre of the cornea to the retina just below the optic papilla, is only 40 mm. The upper measurement (45 mm) applies to close vision with the head raised. Normal distant vision is obtained when the head is held at normal level, with the ray of light passing through the centre of the cornea and impinging upon the centre of the retina. Distant objects would be viewed most effectively with the head depressed and the light ray striking the retina low down in the eye.

According to Walls in *The Vertebrate Eye*, horses (and sheep) have no powers of accommodation other than that provided by a ramp retina. The cornea of the horse is very tough and strong and very inelastic. The sclerotic coat is thick at its rim where it embraces the cornea but it thins down immediately external to the corneal margin so that the sclera below this point acquires a bluish tint, imparted to it by the vessels of the underlying choroid coat. The sclera has another function in addition to affording support to the eyeball and its contents and this is to ensure that the distances from cornea to the back of the eyeball will remain constant in order that the vision may not be impaired at various focal distances.

Without the rigidity provided by the sclerotic coat, the squeezing effect set up by the eyelids and oculo-motor muscles, attached to and surrounding the eyeball, would result in lengthening the eyeball and this would put focusing completely out of order. In some species of vertebrates, notably some of the fishes, the sclera is reinforced by bony tubes, known as *ossicles*, which give additional rigidity to the scleral walls. When we come to the chapter dealing with fishes, we shall read more about these structures and how they work.

The cornea in the horse may be regarded as ovoid, or egg-shaped in its horizontal direction, with the wide end of the egg on the nasal side and the narrow end on the temporal side. The disparity may be as much as 3–5 mm. The border of the cornea of the horse carries two eccentric, grey or white curved areas from 2–3 mm in width, which are most evident in old subjects. They are not present in foals and may not appear before the third year, after which they increase in density every year. The shape and condition of the cornea is most important and any irregularity in its contour will give rise to distortion of the visual image. This produces what is known as *astigmatism*.

Horses are naturally astigmatic, the cornea being rather more convex in one direction than in the other. Seals and most amphibious mammals share the condition, though it is of little account in animals attempting to see under water, but of some consequence in purely terrestrial animals. The cornea under water has a refractive index identical with that of its surroundings.

A point often overlooked is the fact that the volume of the eye and the fullness of curvature within the cornea may exhibit seasonal variations. In spring and summer this may be evident, while in lean times and wintry weather the cornea may appear less curved and the intraocular pressure may temporarily fall.

THE IRIS

The iris is characteristic of that seen in equines collectively, and in some ruminants, in having hanging from its upper edge, three or four pigmented projections known as the corpora nigra. These are suspended at the upper edge of the pupillary orifice and a lesser number (usually) will project upwards from the lower rim of the iris. Altogether, these occlude a considerable portion of the aperture of the pupil. It is unlikely, however, that their presence has any injurious effect on vision. By experimenting with a camera, using similar projections attached to the edge of the diaphragmatic orifice, a negligible effect upon the image is observable.

These corpora nigra originated as outgrowths from the black, pigmented layer lying at the posterior surface of the iris. In the young horse, the pupil is round, but between the fifth and sixth years of life, the shape of the pupil becomes elliptical in the transverse direction. The pupil in the horse, in company with other animals, dilates in a dim light but also when its oxygen supply is reduced. A horse's pupils dilate, therefore, when it is galloped.

THE CRYSTALLINE LENS

This varies in shape a great deal in different species, especially regarding its size compared with that of the eyeball and its general shape. Nicolas gave the absolute volume of the lens in cubic centimetres, as 3·2 in the horse, 2·2 in the ox, 0·7 in the pig and 0·5 in the dog and cat. In man the proportion of the lens to the eyeball is 1:18; in the horse 1:16·3, and in the dog 1:10·2.

During the embryonic development of animals the lens is surrounded by a network of blood vessels. These normally become absorbed by the time of birth. The rat is somewhat exceptional in this respect as the vessels do not disappear completely but persist through life as a pattern of network crossing the pupil.

In the horse, as in most of the carnivora and ungulates, the size of the lens is always proportionate to the requirements of the animal with respect to its environment, and its light requirements. In many individual instances the horse lens shows a yellowish discolouration, as it grows older. This also occurs in the human lens during advancing years, but is not in any way connected with a need for colour filtration. A protein breakdown within the lens and the interaction of protamin and cysteine results in the formation of melanin, which does not in any way help vision.

In the growing foal, the lens is practically round, reddish and cloudy. In consequence, a foal absorbs practically 10 per cent of the blue light entering its eye, whilst an adult horse absorbs about 85 per cent. The lens of the foal is surrounded by a close network of blood vessels whose disappearance is slow. In the adult horse one should be able to observe with an ophthalmoscope, membranous particles and filaments in the vitreous, these being the unabsorbed walls of blood vessels and debris.

In most adult horses the absorption and disappearance of the hyaloid artery has become virtually complete. The hyaloid artery feeds the vitreous substance during its development. It enters the eye at the optic papilla and extends to the posterior surface of the lens. After absorption of the arterial walls, a canal is left in the vitreous. In the dog this is very fine but in the horse it may be 2·3 mm in diameter and can be seen with suitable lighting in the horse's eye, sometimes with the help of an ophthalmoscope, but more readily in the dead eye after suitable methods of staining have been adopted, as with fluorescein.

In both horse and dog, retention of part of the hyaloid artery may be associated with the development of a posterior polar cataract.

THE EYELIDS

In the horse, the eyelids are fine and close-fitting. The upper eyelid is the thicker and both lids are thinnest at the temporal canthus. The upper eyelid carries a number of stiff eyelashes in four rows. The lashes cross each other but do not interlace. In the lower lids only a few thin straggly hairs can be seen. In both the upper and lower lids most of the lashes emerge from the central part of the lid and only a few from the extremities.

In the horse, as in the dog, a regular row of black dots lie closely approximated to the upper lid, immediately behind the lashes. Each is a miniature sebaceous gland with a central tubule which discharges a lubricant onto the edges of the lids. In the horse there may be 40–50 of these structures, which are known as Meibomian glands. The two lids surround the opening known as the *palpebral fissure*.

THE TAPETUM

The horse has a tapetum behind the retina. It consists of two parts: The *tapetum lucidum* situated below the papilla may be yellow, yellowish, green, yellowish blue or multicoloured. Sometimes the colouring differs in the two eyes. The tapetal stars may be seen through an ophthalmoscope as being green or blue, situated in the middle of a larger, lighter coloured spot.

The *tapetum nigrum* is the part of the membrane situated above the papilla. It may be green or blue or purplish-brown, or brick-red interspersed with bands of chocolate. The papilla itself is elliptical, occasionally almost circular, and it lies in the temporal region surrounded by pigmented tapetum nigrum. Its blood vessels, unlike those in the dog, which enter through the middle of the papilla, emerge through the outer periphery of it. Instead of being long and tree-like, as in the dog, they reach only a short distance into the retina and sometimes can hardly be detected below the papilla. The branches are about 25 in number.

In the ass and mule the tapetum is similar, but as the cornea in these animals is situated a little higher in the optic globe than in the horse, the papilla appears to be nearer the centre of the retina and is therefore easier to find with the ophthalmoscope. In the eye of the horse the ophthalmoscope has to be turned *downwards* towards the fundus of the eye to pick out the tapetum.

THE MEMBRANA NICTITANS

In the horse, this is very easily raised into full view by gentle pressure on the lower eyelid. In an animal developing tetanus the third eyelid almost permanently covers the retracted eye from a very early stage of the disease; sometimes one or two days before the generalised muscular tetany becomes obvious.

ACCOMMODATION

The horse, like some fish, (the ray and members of the skate family) is dependent almost wholly upon the ramp retina to obtain a useful degree of focus. The principle involved is that the retina has an uneven slope so that the distance from the cornea to the retina varies regularly. When the horse was more in use than it is today, several observers decided that all horses were not only astigmatic but also either myopic (short-sighted), or hypermetropic (long-sighted).

The discrepancy arose from the fact that the ramp retina gives a different impression according to whether the man behind the ophthalmoscope is 5 ft 5 in, or 6 ft 2 in in height. To make matters even more complicated, it makes a considerable difference in the reading whether the observer is dealing with a twelve-hand pony, or a seventeen-hand horse.

The explanation is that to get a correct reading from a ramp retina, one must cause the light from the ophthalmoscope to pass exactly through the centre of the cornea and land upon the exact centre of the optic disc. Any deviation from this angle, directed either upward or downward will give a different result.

In a normal horse with a normal eye, the distance from the centre of the cornea to the papilla is 40 mm. From the centre of the cornea to the centre of the retina it is 43 mm. The distance from the centre of the cornea to a spot on the retina above the cornea centre, but equidistant from the papilla, is 45 mm. Whatever the height of the observer, his eye must be level with the centre of the cornea when he makes his observation. If above it, he looks down to find the papilla. If below it, he will either not find it at all, or he will be looking upwards through the eye and getting a false measurement.

The next matter to consider when we are endeavouring to determine how much and how far a horse can see, is eye placement, and what obstacles are introduced by eye position, width of forehead and muzzle, and the position of the head in relation to the horse's body at any given moment. In Thoroughbreds with fairly narrow foreheads, the eyes will be directed obliquely outwards at an angle possibly of 30 degrees, with a line drawn from the poll, down the centre of the face. In a broad-faced Shire, the angle might be as much as 40 degrees, with a much wider foreface lying between eyes and ground.

Two certainties arise out of these findings. The first is that even if the Thoroughbred may see objects at a distance with two eyes converging upon them simultaneously (which is when both ears become pricked forward); it is certain that it will be unable to converge upon any object four feet or less in front of its eyes. This implies that no show jumper can see the obstacle in front of it at any distance under four feet, or can only see it with one eye at a time, if it is given free rein and allowed to tilt its head slightly sideways. In a steeplechase, or a hurdle race, the horse propels itself upwards when about six feet from the fence or hurdle, and trusts to the *vis a tergo* developed by momentum, to carry it over the jump. Any show jumper that approaches a six-foot wall, loses all sight of it unless it can make its leap at about six feet from the jump; and when we realise that the horse is approaching the jump at a speed of 16 yards per second, it is obvious that the calculation of the height and nature of the jump must be made when the horse is at least 16 yards from the jump. The take-off, if it is not to be a blind jump, must be made not nearer than six feet from the obstacle.

The horse lands on one fore foot, then on the other, and the eye should be able to see the ground, at least the point upon which the second foot will land. This too can occur only when the eyes of the horse are at least four feet from the ground when the horse is coming down, with head carried low. It is safer to assume that the horse *never* sees the landing ground, and at the time of impact of the fore feet in succession, with the ground, his head is being raised again, probably with the assistance of the bit and reins.

The only time that a horse can converge upon objects a short distance ahead, is when the head is *raised*, or when it is held *close to the ground*. A horse grazing in a field with head down, can see all around itself by looking between its own knees and hocks.

The horse enters the ring with its head held level and with the front line of head and muzzle perpendicular with the ground. Rays of light then pass through the cornea and land on the retina, its central part. These rays are at a focal length of 43 mm. If the horse raises its head to look at the clapping spectators in the stands, the

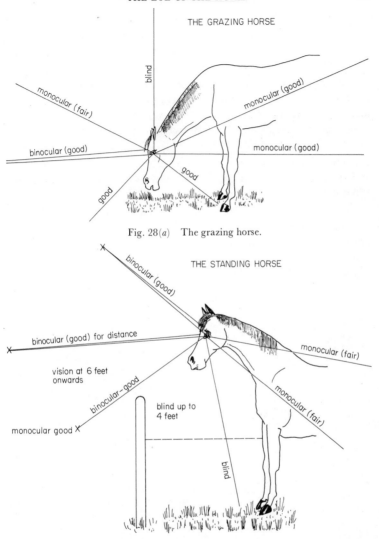

Fig. 28(a)   The grazing horse.

Fig. 28(b)   The standing horse.

rays of light will strike the retina near the optic disc at a focal length of 40 mm. If it looks down at the ground at the approach to the jump the rays will enter the lower part of the cornea and fall upon the upper third of the retina at a focal length of 45 mm. This presumes that the horse enjoys a certain amount of freedom of head movement without too rigid use of the martingale. If a horse is to perform to the greatest advantage, whether in the jumping ring, the racecourse or the show-ring, it *must* be free, so far as is possible, to select its own head position.

The horse was provided with a long flexible neck for several reasons. One is that in a state of nature its head *had* to reach down to the ground for grazing. Another was to maintain balance by using the head as a pendulum, or as a bobweight. The third was to enable it to use its eyes. With the help of a flexible neck the horse is enabled, in spite of difficulties presented by the width of its head and the breadth of its muzzle, to see through an angle greater than 180 degrees.

In the ass, the forehead is wider and the neck shorter and less flexible than in the horse. The ass, however, enjoys far better posterior vision and can kick an object, such as a dog, three feet behind its own hindquarters, without bending its neck or turning its head.

CHAPTER 7

VISION IN OTHER MAMMALS

OTHER UNGULATES

The earliest members of the ox and deer family possessed horns and open orbits but apparently the combination was not a suitable one and in the course of evolution they developed the closed orbit for protection. The smaller deer and a few of the larger, including the moose, retain the open orbit but these do not fight seriously with horns, they are usually content with an interlacing and pushing technique.

In the ruminants the anterior portion of the retina is usually the larger and this enables the cow to see her own flanks whilst her head is carried forward, which incidentally allows her an excellent opportunity to kick her milker. In the Highland breed of cattle, for instance, their deeply-set eyes and masses of overhanging hair, enable them to see very little upon which their eyes can converge. It is generally believed that the bull closes its eyes when it charges, which may have a bearing upon the relatively high rate of survival of matadors. Like the horse, the bull is completely colour blind so the traditional red cloak is used more for appearance than for effect and would be quite as efficient if it were black.

The cow, however, is not quite so considerate, as she charges with her eyes wide open and also follows every twist and turn of her victim, with the greatest of ease and accuracy, another proof that the female of the species is more deadly than the male.

In the ox the membrana nictitans is a thick membrane and contains folds. Animals such as horses, cattle and deer, among many others, possess the ability to detect moving objects *behind* their own bodies. In a race, even if the jockey cannot see what follows close behind him, his mount can. It employs the rods situated at the nasal (anterior) quadrant of the retina. Horses raced in blinkers can see only straight ahead.

Whatever position the head assumes, whether held high or low, the eyes of cattle always remain horizontal. When feeding with head to

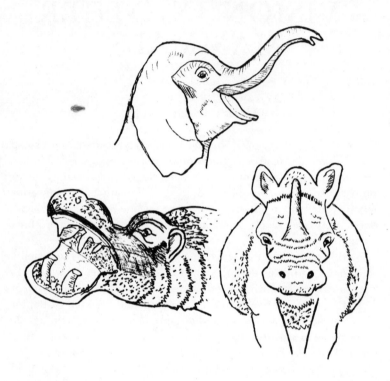

Fig. 29   The largest animals have the smallest eyes.

ground, the eyes are directed forwards and slightly upwards. Cattle possess a triangular tapetum.

While we are discussing ungulates, we may introduce certain large animals, such as the elephant, rhinoceros, hippopotamus and whale. It is noteworthy that as a rule the larger the animal, or the larger its head, the smaller is the eye relative to the size of the head. This applies to all the foregoing large mammals. Their visual acuity is generally poor.

THE ELEPHANT

Among all the large mammals the elephant has probably the smallest eye in proportion to its body size. Although provided with tusks it still has an open orbit, perhaps because the tusks represent teeth, not horns. As a rule eye movement and intelligence go together, but nobody could accuse an elephant of being dim-witted, although it has practically no eye movement.

It is unable to close its eyelids tightly and has no special retina adaptation to day or night vision. The eye is furnished with rods but not so well with cones. It possesses a tapetum so it must be presumed its nocturnal vision is satisfactory.

By day it has been said that the elephant's vision would compare unfavourably with that of a Pekinese dog. Apparently it sees all its needs. A large, bulky animal, nobody's prey, has less need for acuity of vision than one likely to be eaten. One may imagine they see close objects reasonably well but in the wild state they appear to hear better than they see. The notice boards displayed in parts of Africa, advising giving priority on the roads to wild elephants seems to indicate this. These animals have no conception of colour at all.

THE RHINOCEROS

This is another animal of huge size with an extraordinarily small eye, together with very low visual acuity. The eyes are almost hidden and the eyelids blink very rapidly; so much so before it charges that the movement of the lids cannot be seen.

Like other large animals the rhinoceros is colour blind.

THE HIPPOPOTAMUS

The brows are arched in such a way that when the whole body and most of the head are submerged, the eyes will remain above water level, together with the nostrils. This is characteristic of animals, including the frogs, which like to live in water but are unable to see through it when the eyes are submerged. The pupil is an oval, horizontal aperture. The eyes themselves are very small.

Among other large animals we must include the whale.

THE WHALE

The head of the whale constitutes one third of the whole body. Although the whale lives entirely in water, it nevertheless carries the mammalian eye, and like that in all the larger animals, this is very small. It may be regarded as immovable so that the whale depends upon head and neck movements. The tiny eyes lie far back in its enormous head and are directed downwards and outwards. The whale sees practically nothing when its eyes are above water level, and as it cannot move them, it seems likely that it comes to the surface only to breathe and blow. It can close the eyes only with

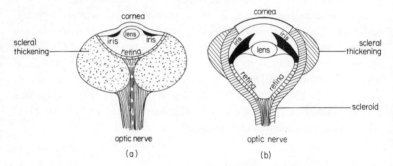

Fig. 30   (a)   Eye of the whale. Note the very thick scleral thickenings.
          (b)   Eye of the seal. The seal has a spherical pupil and a slit iris which provides a stenopaic pupil when the animal is on land. It appears to be able to focus nearby objects on the ground at a matter of twelve feet when on land.

difficulty, if at all, and seldom for more than a few seconds, so apparently the whale sleeps with eyes open.

The Toothless Whales (Baleen Whales) *can* close their eyes, but they secrete an oil which protects them from the water. Oil also replaces tears and waterproofs the cornea. All the accessory glands around the eye also secrete oil.

The eye is seldom larger than a medium-sized orange, but it is packed inside a very large and thick pressure-resisting casing which encircles the lower part of the eyeball. The elephant has a rather similar scleral thickening. Without the rigidity provided by this sclerotic thickening, the squeezing effect of the eyelids and the muscles would result in lengthening the eyeball with distortion of vision.

THE SEAL

In these animals we find a somewhat thickened sclera, but unlike that in the whales, it is not continued back to the hinder part of the eye but forms a protective ring just behind the corneal margin.

The seal has an open orbit resembling that in the dog and cat. It makes excellent use of what might commonly be regarded as a visual defect to obtain clear vision on land, for in daylight its pupil becomes a vertical slit. The seal is also a victim of astigmatism in company with most amphibious animals, but as the direction of the astigmatism is exactly opposite to that of the slit pupil so as to cross one another, it will result in producing something akin to a pinhole camera, and in bright daylight the need for any other method of accommodation becomes unnecessary. The cornea of the seal has the same refractive index as the sea water so the astigmatism can be disregarded under water. The seal has also a useful ciliary muscle so that it can regulate its accommodation if need be, in the usual manner. In the seal, as in the sea lion, the size of the pupil can be regulated voluntarily.

Compared with those of other sizeable aquatic animals the eyes of the seal are fairly large, and as the seals depend upon catching numbers of small fishes, the eyes require a wide optical angle to keep these in view. The eyes move only a little in their sockets but seals have flexible necks and under water can gyrate like a fish and get a clear view of everything in the vicinity. The eyes are directed slightly upwards so that floating on the water surface the seal can search the rocks overhead before making a landing. This may also be why performing seals can catch fish thrown to them and balance balls on their noses.

The seal sees what is happening on land or rocks from the water and on the way to a beach, will often lift its body halfway out of the water fifty yards from the shore, to inspect the landscape for possible danger, or a mother seal may behave similarly when seeking out her cub left on the beach.

CHAPTER 8

VISION IN BIRDS

THE EYES OF BIRDS

In a number of their species, birds possess a very highly developed visual sense combined with the ability to recognise colour. They even make use of this as a means of sex recognition, although in the avian world it is the male that enjoys the thrills associated with personal

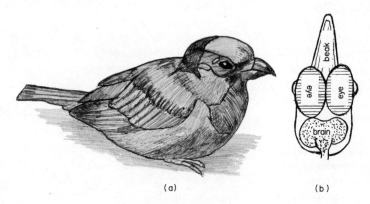

(a)   (b)

Fig. 31   (a)   Eye of a sparrow as it appears in life.
          (b)   Eye of a sparrow in section. The eyeball occupies
the greater part of the head, the brain occupies a much smaller
                           part.

adornment. Not only do birds recognise the sex of their associates by the colour of their plumes but they also recognise their enemies and rivals. Fortunately, in birds fashions do not change, and in this respect when distinguishing between the sexes they have the advantage over mere man.

Birds, except at mating time, are seldom antagonistic creatures

96

and in their everyday lives, their main necessity is an ability to take rapid flight when danger threatens. Their safety depends upon keen vision. The eyeballs of birds when compared with the visible eye are immensely large and occupy a considerable proportion of the entire head, leaving little room for brain or eye muscles.

Although few birds are able to move their eyes (gulls are an exception), they are provided with long, flexible necks which permit

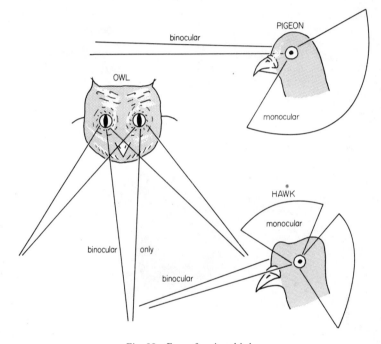

Fig. 32   Eyes of various birds.

free and wide movement of the head into remarkable positions. The owl, for example, is devoid of eye movement but it can turn its head round until it is facing the tail, or it can throw the head back until it is completely upside-down.

Any bird which spends its time mainly in the air seeking its food from the ground far below, needs a special kind of eye. So does one that is half-blind by day and catches its prey during the hours of near-darkness.

Soaring at several hundred feet above a woodland pasture, a hawk has to recognise its prey, then swoop down upon it. Several seconds may elapse during the downward dive and the mouse the hawk viewed will by then be yards away from its original point of location. Accordingly, the hawk has to swoop with eyes wide open, registering during its rapid descent, every move made by the mouse.

An owl, on the other hand, has little need of diurnal vision, in spite of the fact that the Tawny owl may sometimes be seen hunting hedgerows in broad daylight. This owl has ear openings differing in

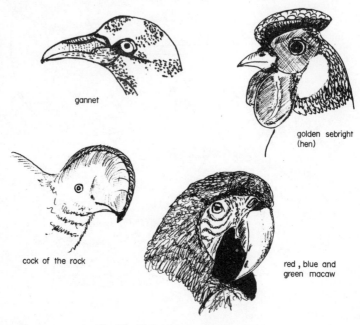

gannet

golden sebright
(hen)

cock of the rock

red , blue and
green macaw

Fig. 33   Birds with monocular vision only.

size and shape, adapted for accurate location of the prey. Few other owls have any useful diurnal vision.

Some of the birds, particularly those with 'waisted' or bell-shaped eyes, or eyes that are pear-shaped with a central constriction, are strengthened in extraordinary fashion. In the owls, for example, the sclera is so impregnated with bone that in size and shape it may resemble the walls of a pill-box. This ring of thickening is termed the Ringwulst. The majority of birds with laterally placed eyes, (not the owls), make use of monocular vision, bobbing the head from side to side, or up-and-down, in order to see the object first with one eye, then with the other. Usually, directly in front of the

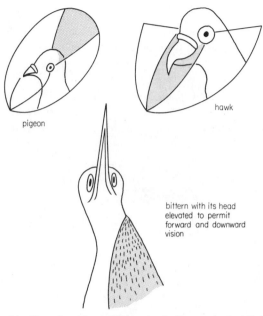

pigeon

hawk

bittern with its head
elevated to permit
forward and downward
vision

Fig. 34   Binocular vision in birds—the shading marks the blind
areas.

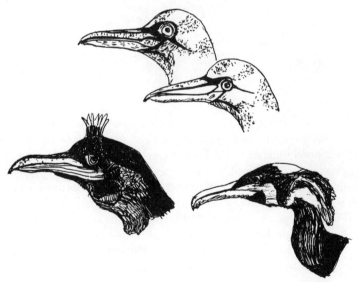

Fig. 35   Common British diving birds—note the 'sighting'
channel down the length of the beak below the eyes.

beak, there is a triangular blindspot, varying in extent according to eye placement and beak and head shape. The domestic hen cannot see the grain in front of her beak so does her dance-like walk among the food particles with nodding head, using single eyes in succession.

Convergence is out of the question in birds with bilateral vision but in many hawks, eagles, and diving birds, there are 'sights', or guide lines, from eye to beak, which enable the bird to take aim at

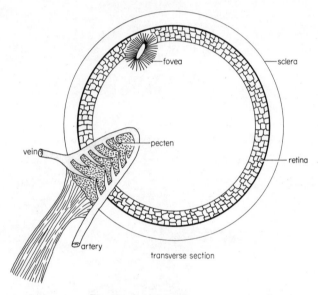

Fig. 36   An avian pecten.

its prey. Such birds can also converge when they are in the air and the head can be hung downwards. In this position a wide surface of the ground hundreds of feet below can be viewed quite accurately. As previously mentioned, the owls can turn their heads completely around on their necks, or can turn the head backwards until it faces the wrong direction. What need, then, is there for eye movement?

Birds, such as the snipe and other waders in which the eyes are set low-down in the face, are able to turn their heads, mounted on long flexible necks, in any direction. This enables two laterally-placed eyes to be used alternately. It must be remembered that birds, whether like the snipe on the ground with beak buried in the soil or up in the air like larks or swallows, have to be able to keep

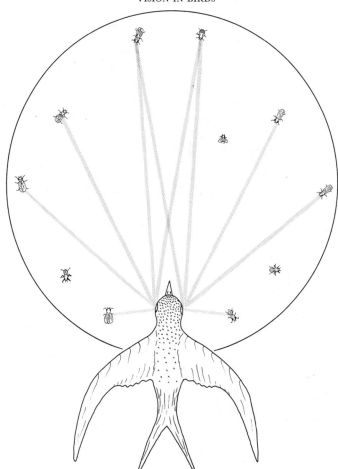

Fig. 37 An insectivorous bird, such as a swallow, whilst in search of flies in the air, uses the temporal and central foveae in each eye to provide excellent binocular vision. Simultaneously, by using each eye separately to view objects laterally situated, it secures excellent monocular vision.

constant watch overhead, which is the danger point. The snipe, with no eye movement, can contract its soft lens within the aperture of the pupil, until it bulges out into the anterior chamber of the eye, and can transmit an impression from any quarter to its brain.

Birds vary, not only in the shape of their eyeballs, but also in their internal structure. Most birds have in their retinae two adjuncts to visual acuity. One is the presence of *foveae*, hypersensitive areas conveying an immense number of cones; and also what is known as the pecten.

The domestic pigeon, as such, has lost its foveae, but how greatly this applies to, or affects vision in homing birds is uncertain. The so called 'eye-sign' used by fanciers in selecting homers, may possibly be associated with the presence or absence of foveae.

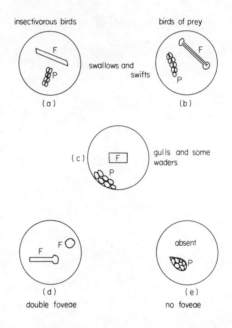

Fig. 38   The retina in some birds. F = fovea; P = pecten.

The appearance of the foveae varies in different bird families. The common form is a narrow band. This is especially the case in the insect eaters, in which it is elongated so that head movements will be less if the bird is to keep a moving insect under observation. In the woodpigeon it is shallow and variable. In the tame, domestic pigeons it is usually absent. In birds of prey there are usually two separate foveae, each of which may be centred on a different object.

Fast flying birds such as swallows and swifts which catch minute insects in the air during flight need exceptional vision, nearly all have double foveae. Seabirds and the waders have a single fovea which is exceptionally wide. When double foveae are present, the temporal fovea views objects straight ahead while the central fovea takes in lateral vision.

Birds see objects on either side of their bodies better than those straight ahead. This is particularly helpful in birds like starlings which fly very fast, in packed flocks.

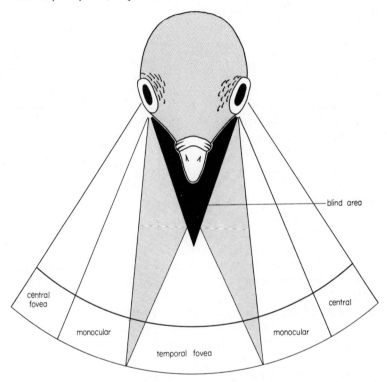

Fig. 39   Pigeon vision.

Birds of prey do not depend too greatly upon the temporal fovea but turn their heads rapidly from side to side to keep a moving prey in constant view. Night birds, the owls, nightjars and others, have no use for a macula and depend upon rods rather than upon cones. Gannets, which drop sometimes a hundred feet to pick up their fish from the sea, have no fovea.

In birds the retina possesses another feature. This is the pecten which is a pleated fin of pigmented, highly vascular tissue, which projects through the vitreous body in the direction of the lens. It provides a supplementary blood supply to the retina and is present

E

in all birds, including night fliers. The pecten is a development of the blood vessels coming through the optic nerve to the retina. In mammals, these spread over the surface of the retina like the branches of a tree. In birds they rise from the optic disc like the pages of a book, and are believed to improve visual acuity, though their real purpose seems to be to feed the retina.

The foveae in birds are usually placed laterally as temporal foveae, and also centrally, arranged on a band. They provide not only lateral and, less often, frontal vision, but enable the bird to see overhead and also behind the head. The central fovea is particularly useful in birds, such as starlings, which fly in regimental order, in flocks, and turn in unison. Such birds, together with the swallows, and the alert and active kingfisher, have a pair of foveae in each eye. When a temporal and central fovea are present in the same bird (diurnal), the temporal fovea is used for viewing objects directly ahead, and the central for viewing objects on either side of the head. In some insectivorous birds the fovea is in band form; in birds of prey, swallows and swifts it is represented by a pair of pinholes at the end of the band.

Let us now consider the eyeball in birds and how it is constructed:

There are four shapes of eyes. The first is the tubular type, somewhat pear-shaped, with a wide retina and a much smaller, semi-spherical, protruding cornea. The owl has this kind of eye. Four-fifths of it will be hidden within the skull and only the front of the cornea will show. The scleral ossicle is very obvious.

The second type is seen in the domestic hen; an eye, flattened from front to back, to an oval shape.

In the birds of prey, the hawks for example, the eyeball is bell-shaped with the cornea protruding, but much less in diameter than in the owl.

In the small songbirds, the cornea is a little flattened but more nearly spherical.

Birds have kept their third eyelids and many, particularly the owls, use them as a protection against the summer glare. A few have a transparent window in some portion of the third eyelid and birds on migration close their third eyelids during long flights.

Shags and cormorants make use of this window when swimming beneath the surface of the water. With the lid closed, either of these can chase a fish swimming at a distance of ten feet from the bird's head, at which range it can see the fish and keep it in focus.

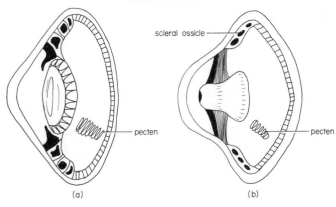

scleral ossicle

pecten

pecten

(a) (b)

Fig. 40   The eyes of a bird in section. The tubular eye of an owl, showing how it overcomes the problem of accommodation. As shown in (a) the unaccommodated eye is able to deal with the distant vision. In (b) the soft elastic lens is gripped by the surrounding ciliary body and squeezed into a pear shape, providing for close-up vision. The object growing from the retina is the pecten. Its purpose is to increase the bloodflow to the retina; to bring it oxygen and remove waste products.

Gannets watch a shoal of fish from a great height, take aim along their hanging beaks, and drop. With any luck they will transfix a fish.

In birds, as well as in frogs, alligators and turtles, there is no retractor muscle operating the eyeball, and the third eyelid is operated by a muscle with a long tendon working through a loop, which acts as a pulley. In birds that possess scleral ossicles the wall of the eye is protected during the act of accommodation. This is effected by squeezing the soft lens within the orifice of the pupil and lengthening the lens and distorting its shape until it produces a sharp retinal image. This imposes a deal of pressure upon the scleral wall. The pupil in the bird's iris can be operated voluntarily, unlike that in mammals which responds only to the influence of light and darkness.

A swallow or a hawk will converge its eyes until the central and temporal foveae come into operation. The bird will probably see three images simultaneously: one ahead and one on either side. It is likely its brain is attuned to converting these into a single, concerted picture. House sparrows can see at least twenty-five yards and chaffinches probably further than this. The robin is in a class of its own. It is able to see all around its body at one time; or directly ahead, using both eyes simultaneously; or it can adopt monocular vision and observe objects on one side of its head only. A cock robin can see a female and recognise her sex at thirty yards. On the other hand it can be deceived by a tiny piece of red rag stuffed between the branches of a garden bush, and will attack it furiously.

CHAPTER 9

THE EYES OF FISHES

Fishes have certain advantages over other animals. One lies in the possession of the 'lateral line' by many species, which provides information regarding the relationship of the body to surrounding objects or obstacles, a proprioceptive capacity, comparable in some ways with the radar perception in bats.

Fishes, too, possess a colour sense, as may be implied from the mating displays of fish living in shallow water. See Smythe: *The Haunts and Habits of Fishes*.

As one descends below the surface farther and farther, the light becomes more dim and at great depths gives way to complete darkness because all available light has been absorbed within the surface layers. Plants cannot grow in very deep waters unless they can float near the surface. In these areas fish carry their own lamps and it is to be presumed that other fish can interpret their purpose and meaning. Such areas of illumination are built into the bodies of the fishes.

The refractive index of the cornea of the fish is similar to that of water. so in passing from water to cornea the rays of light are bent to a lesser degree than in passing from air to cornea. Consequently, the corneal surface in a fish can be flatter than that in a land animal or mammal. In Analeps, the 'Four-eyed Fish', the iris passes across the eye as a horizontal bar which divides the pupil into above-water and below-water sections, which the fish can utilise when floating on the surface of the water. The Archer fish spits drops of water at flies near the surface and brings them down on the water.

Fishes, like birds, are frequently provided in front of their eyes with steering sights in the form of lines or ridges which enable them to take aim. In deep water the pressure upon an unguarded cornea might be excessive and in consequence many fish wear solid 'spectacles'. The Norwegian bream is a striking example. Spectacles take the place of eyelids although one variety of grey mullet has 'fatty eyelids'. Eyes wearing spectacles remain permanently wide open. A space exists between cornea and spectacle to allow eye movement.

Sharks, particularly the basking shark and the whale shark, have especially thick eye casings but not comparable with those of the

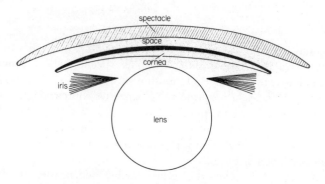

Fig. 41   The spectacle of a fish shown in section.

sperm whale, which are much thicker, in spite of the fact that sharks dive far deeper than whales.

In deep-sea fishes many of the eyes are tubular and employ something after the fashion of a ramp retina; the retina is arranged so that through a spherical lens, it provides several focal lengths. See Fig. 42 (a) and (b). In the bony fishes the lens is also spherical, much like a marble in shape, and the iris may be present or absent, and the ciliary muscle is also missing. In its place is a special retractor muscle of the lens. This normally rests against the hinder surface of the cornea at which position it supplies close-range vision. When the fish needs a rather longer range (distance vision is limited below the surface), it contracts this muscle and pulls the lens back from the cornea.

Opposed to this is the more rounded eye of the shark, in which a distinct iris exists and the muscle is positioned so that it pulls the lens *forward*. In the sharks, a gelatinous ring surrounds the lens and the sclera is considerably thickened. In some fishes the eye is irregularly triangular in shape, so that the light passing downwards

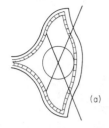
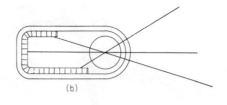

Fig. 42   More eyes of fishes.
(a)   The ramp retina found in skate and rays. In principle it is much like the horse; light rays enter above or below.
(b)   The tubular eye seen in fishes that live at great depths. Also on the ramp principle but designed to withstand considerable pressure.

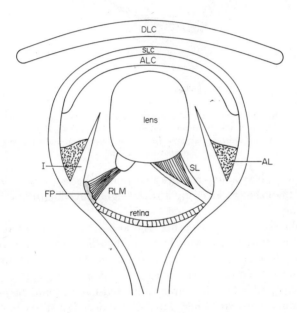

Fig. 43   The eye of a Bony Fish (Teleost), in section.
DLC = spectacle; SLC = scleral layer of cornea; ALC = true cornea; AL = annular ligament; FP = falciform process; SL = suspensory ligament of lens; RLM = retractor muscle of lens; I = iris.

The lens rests against the cornea for close-up vision and is drawn back by the retractor muscle for distant vision (probably up to fifteen feet).

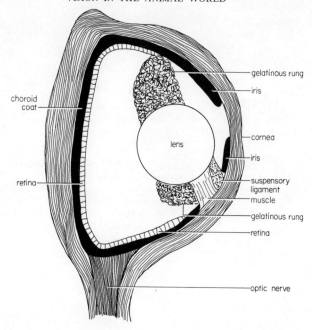

Fig. 44 Section of the eye of a shark. Muscle = the muscle
which pulls the eye forward, not backward as in most fishes (Protractor lentis); gelatinous rung = cartilage surrounding and
supporting the lens.

through a spherical lens reaches a portion of the retina closer in focal
length than that received by a ray of light travelling in an upward
direction.

In some of the deep sea fishes, and also in the squid, the rods and
cones are arranged at varying levels, so that the image can recede and
advance through the whole range of vision. This removes any need
for muscular or other means of accommodation.

In nearly all bony fishes three kinds of visual cells may be present:
rods, cones and twin cones. Most of the deep sea fishes have only
single cones. The double cones are found in those fish which swim
and feed near the surface and have to withstand what to them must
be bright illumination.

Pollack, rockfish and shads are all provided with double cones
only. Even surface feeders living far out in the ocean are similarly
furnished. Mackerel, the mullet family, tunny-fish and curiously,
flatfish also carry a number of twin cones. One would imagine that

flatfish which live near the bottom, would not be included, although most flatfish favour comparatively shallow water with a sandy bottom. Even though many are taken by dredgers it is known that flatfish haunt sandbanks and mudbanks which become exposed at low tide, or are at that time close to the surface of the sea. A curious feature respecting flatfish was noticed by me while fishing for bass in the Yealm Estuary, from a pier at high tide, in ten feet of often very rough water. Using a small spinning bait kept close to the surface, I frequently landed a good-sized flounder, which, lying on the seabottom or near it, was able to see and rise for a bait drawn fairly rapidly through the water, at least seven feet above its head. In the flatfishes the pupil contracts from a heart-shaped opening to a narrow crescent.

The lateral eyes of most fishes make it impossible for the fish to see more of its body than its tail. This probably explains why the lateral line is useful.

The lateral line is a fluid-filled tube or canal lying just below the skin but visible through it. It communicates with the water by a series of minute pores. The canal is lined with nerve endings which are responsive to water vibrations and convey information to the brain regarding the position of the fish and the nature of its environment. Even in very muddy water when the vision is impaired the use of the lateral line enables the fish to move freely without collision.

The flatfishes have a regular eye cycle. Each commences as an ordinary little fish, shaped like a baby mackerel and swimming like one, with an eye on each side of the head. When a month old the baby flatfish settles on the sea bed. It is now white underneath and dark on top. An uneven growth now occurs so that the eye, originally underneath, moves 'round the corner' until both eyes lie on top of the head. The dorsal fin will by now have advanced in a forward direction and prevented the eye's retreat.

Looking upwards towards the light, the flatfish can see a reflection of the seabed in a circle of light overhead, providing the sea is calm and the water not over fifteen feet deep. The flatfish cannot close its eyes and its body colour adjusts itself to that of the sea bed, when it is probable the fish no longer sees itself in the reflection. Other fishes usually have their eyes directed downwards. The most amazing eye placement is in the Hammer-headed shark which has a head shaped as a semicircle with one eye at each end of the radius. (See Fig. 59.)

E*

Flying fishes, it is said, have their eyes directed downwards so that they may look out for enemies below water. It is doubtful, though, whether they see anything through flat corneae, when airborne.

In the skate family a ramp retina, like that of the horse, though a little more exaggerated, is in use.

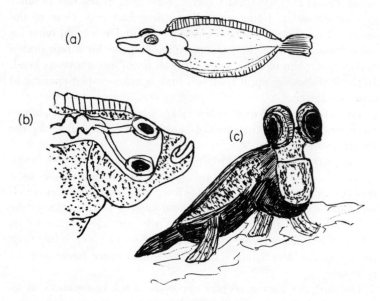

Fig. 45   (a)   A young flatfish. The eyes are sited one on either side of the head and the little fish swims in an upright position. As it grows, one eye 'comes round the corner'.

(b)   Head of a plaice dissected to show decussation of optic nerves and the brain.

(c)   The little mud skipper, only 1½ inches long, has eyes which revolve in all directions within turrets.

In fishes, the compound lens seen in mammals, is replaced by one of simple type since the refractive index of the cornea of the fish is similar to that of water, and only the lens itself comes into operation.

In the bony fishes the cornea is usually elliptical and wider in the horizontal direction. The centre of the cornea is often nearer the nasal angle, thus enlarging the binocular field.

Sharks, skates and rays, as well as most of the bony fishes are provided with round pupils. In the sharks, eels and flat fishes the pupils are contractile. In the sharks the pupil contracts to a diagonal or horizontal slit. It is recognised by skin divers that if one comes face to face with a shark and its pupils contract in this fashion, that the shark means business, and it is wise to surface.

Some fishes have a head shape which favours binocular vision: sharks, pike and trout are examples. It is said that these fish see only objects, or baits, suspended immediately in front of them. This may apply to artificial baits but most fish can smell, through water, and they certainly taste, as they quickly discard most artificial baits taken in the mouth—if able so to do.

As in other animals which hunt or are hunted, eye placement varies in fishes. Those which hunt smaller fish, have their eyes placed frontally, while those which are hunted have monocular vision with eyes placed laterally. The little mud skipper, only $1\frac{1}{2}$ inches long, has its big eyes set in high turrets, in which the eyes revolve in all directions. It has no neck to move, so the eyes do the work. When resting it retracts its eyes into its head and the skin forming the turrets falls over into folds looking like loose eyelids. The medial eye of the lamprey has already been mentioned.

CHAPTER 10

VISION IN REPTILES AND SOME AQUATIC ANIMALS

In this section we will discuss vision in snakes and lizards, crocodiles and alligators, tortoises, terrapins and turtles. In all of these, vision is of the utmost importance and a dominant sense.

Few of the reptiles enjoy what we would regard as long distance vision. They have excellent eyes and all the apparatus conducive to vision up to what in snakes and lizards we might regard as striking distance; but their vision with regard to objects several yards away is limited and unless the object is capable of movement its observation cannot be relied on. The less aggressive members see very clearly anything edible within reach.

Snakes are very quick strikers and to remain in circulation they have to be, since their vision is better than their timing mechanism. An adder or a cobra strikes *at* the moving object but usually fails to make allowance for the fact that the part aimed at will not be 'there' when the fangs reach the spot. The mongoose will rush repeatedly past a snake, so rapidly that the fangs land *behind* its body. The snake has not been trained on clay pigeons, or would have learned to aim ahead of the target. Lizards are more accurate but their prey is usually less mobile.

Many varieties of snakes, (particularly adders) though not all, adopt the colouring of their environment, not instantaneously, but in course of time. This is why adders in some localities are yellow or green, red, or occasionally, almost black. Their markings remain constant, only the body colour varies. Most snakes have a horny eye-covering or blinking. The eye-coverings are part of the skin and are cast at every moult and replaced when the new skin appears.

In snakes, both eyes are laterally placed and monocular vision is the rule. The snake's neck being continuous with its body and only distinguished with difficulty, permits such rapid and all-embracing head movements that monocular vision offers no obstacle.

The majority of snakes lack foveae, although they occur in lizards. The East Indian long-nosed tree snake has them and although it has to rely upon lateral vision it has the finest vision in the snake family and the keenest distance judgement among living creatures. Its pupil is shaped like a keyhole with the circular opening at the front. The head is streamlined, coming to a point at the mouth end, with a sighting groove from each eye down the length of the face through which with one eye the snake can obtain a clear view of the creature it is about to strike.

Snakes focus their eyes by drawing the iris backwards against the vitreous body which bulges in the direction of the pupil and pushes the lens forward to view objects near at hand. They do this when the snakecharmer wriggles his flute close (but not too close) to their eyes. They are not musically-minded but they watch moving objects. Most snakes have lenses which are not spherical, but flattened. Between the lens and the iris in many reptiles, there is an annular thickening around the lens equator which protects the iris when it squeezes the lens. It is termed the *Ringwulst*.

In the diurnal snakes the lens is deep yellow in colour, while in lizards and frogs it is bright yellow. In the turtle it is red or orange. In the male viper the lens is red, and visible through the pupil. In the female, it is yellow.

LIZARDS

These have most efficient eyes although they appear to disregard objects devoid of movement. They also hear well. It is believed that they see orange, yellow, and possibly green, and red, and appear to favour coloured backgrounds. They have lateral eye placement and their lenses are rounded or conical and surrounded by an annular Ringwulst. Some possess closely-packed and elongated cones in their retinae. Others have pure rod retinae. The fovea in the retina is well marked, fairly deep, and centrally placed. Some have the wall fortified by bony plates.

Lizards have little or no eye movement; although the eye is perfect for close work it is uncertain how they are fitted for distance, and it is unlikely they see still objects over more than a few feet away, though they 'see', (or hear) a *moving* object at a distance of at least six feet.

SLOW WORMS

These are legless lizards with excellent sight although often credited with being blind. They detect the slightest movement in a slug or worm, test its quality with the tongue, then seize and devour it.

CHAMELEONS

This is remarkable for the turret-shaped structure which surmounts the comparatively small eye. These '*eye-housings*' as they are termed,

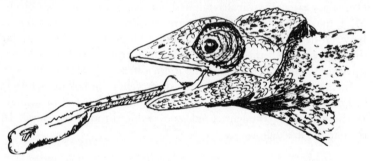

Fig. 46   The chameleon. The eyes are able to move and work independently of one another, although in fishes the movements are in the horizontal plane.

appear to move on swivels. They turn in almost any direction and one eye in its turret can move independently of the other. One eye can be following an insect in front, and the other watching out behind for a potential enemy. Chameleons are slow movers. They stalk their prey by easy stages, then shoot out a tongue of enormous length for the capture.

CROCODILES AND ALLIGATORS

These reptiles enjoy excellent vision on land and fair vision under water. Alligators and crocodiles have both day and night vision and see least during bright sunshine. Both have a third eyelid, or nictitating membrane, with a *central window*.

Crocodiles and alligators both spend the night floating on the surface, or submerged with their eye turrets above water. By day they bask in the sun, often on river banks. Both reptiles are colour blind. The cornea is dome-shaped; the lens thick and flattened, not spherical. The external surface of the eye is constantly lubricated and waterproofed by an oily secretion.

TORTOISES, TERRAPINS AND TURTLES

Tortoises appear (at least) to have some degree of colour vision. Terrapins and turtles feed under water and it is uncertain whether they see colours on land. Their eyes are suited to their separate modes of life. Tortoises undoubtedly have good vision on land. The third eyelid is operated by a muscle and tendon, as in birds. Accommodation is by pressure of the iris upon the vitreous body, which squeezes the lens into the pupil, which is contractile. The eyes of turtles are directed downwards at an angle of 150 degrees, at least when swimming on the surface.

Terrapins appear to have inferior vision as compared with turtles and rely greatly upon sense of smell.

AQUATIC CREATURES, FROGS, TOADS AND NEWTS

Frogs are emmetropic (normally-sighted) on land and strongly hypermetropic (long-sighted) under water. They have little power of accommodation but they are able to push the lens forward and bulge the cornea to obtain a close-up view of a possible victim. Being mainly diurnal they have yellow oil droplets in the retina, but toads, which are mainly nocturnal, have none.

The eyes in frogs and toads have no bony floor in the orbit. The orbits are large and tend to bulge, both in upward and downward direction. When these creatures feed one may take a large worm by one end and commence to swallow it. At each gulp it closes its eyes and pulls them down from their sockets, through the 'missing floor' of the skull into the throat. As they bulge downwards the eyes act as ramrods and push the worm down the throat.

Accommodation is provided by altering the curvature of the lens, as happens in mammals. When the muscles relax, the lens is focused on infinity, and all objects three feet or more from the eyes appear sharp. When the suspensory ligament is relaxed by contraction of the muscle, the lens increases its curvature and objects close at hand can be viewed.

Some varieties of frogs favour the iris propulsion system of accommodation common in reptiles. Newts enjoy equally good vision by day and by night. Salamanders and toads only use their eyes below water during spawning time.

CHAPTER 11

VISION IN INSECTS AND SPIDERS

The visual apparatus and the whole application of vision in insects and the spider family (Araneida) differs greatly from that of the animals which we have already discussed. Responses to light are mediated by (*a*) dermal receptors, (*b*) dorsal ocelli, (*c*) lateral ocelli and (*d*) compound eyes.

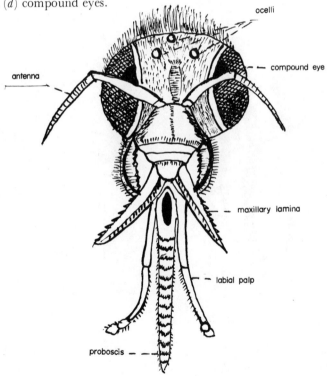

Fig. 47   Head of a Honey Bee.

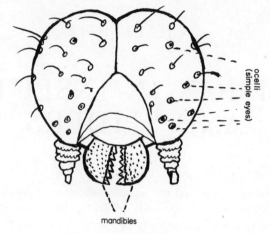

Fig. 48   Head of a caterpillar.

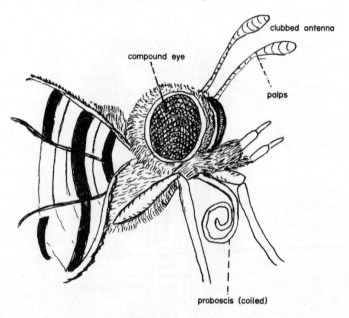

Fig. 49   Head of a butterfly, showing compound eyes.

Several insects, even in the larval form, (some caterpillars for example,) react to light after the ocelli have been covered with opaque material. In the typical insect both compound eyes and ocelli are present, though dorsal ocelli are frequently absent in wingless insects. Lateral ocelli occur in butterflies and a number of other insects. Certain insects possess lateral eyes, the relationship of these to true ocelli is in doubt.

COMPOUND EYES

In these the cornea is divided into a number of separate facets, whereas in an ocellus there is a single facet. Each visual element in a compound eye is known as an ommatidium. The various parts entering into an ommatidium are:

(a) *The cornea:* This consists of a transparent area of cuticle which forms the facet or lens. This is frequently hexagonal.

(b) *The corneagen layer:* This term is applied to the part of the hypodermis lying beneath the cornea.

(c) *The crystalline cone lens:* This is a group of four cells.

(d) *Primary iris cells:* These are densely pigmented cells disposed in a circle surrounding the cells of the crystalline cone and the corneagen layer.

(e) *The retinule:* This represents the basal portion of each ommatidium and is composed of a group of pigmented visual cells, each of the latter being continuous with a post-retinal fibre. Collectively the visual cells secrete an internal optic rod or rhabdom. The portion secreted by each individual cell is termed the rhabdomere. The individual fibres pass through the cell and emerge as a single nerve.

The rhabdom forms the central axis of the retinula and is in direct contact with the extremity of the crystalline cone.

(f) *The secondary iris cells:* These are elongated pigment cells which surround the primary iris cells and the retinula, separating each ommatidium from its neighbours.

Four types of compound eyes are recognised, depending upon the nature of the crystalline cone, whether it be present or absent, and upon its origin. In general terms, the compound eyes develop embryonically. A zone of larval epidermis undergoes cell division and from this the eye develops. Certain cells move towards the base and form the retinulae, while others form the crystalline cone cells. When fully developed, the compound cells of the eyes of

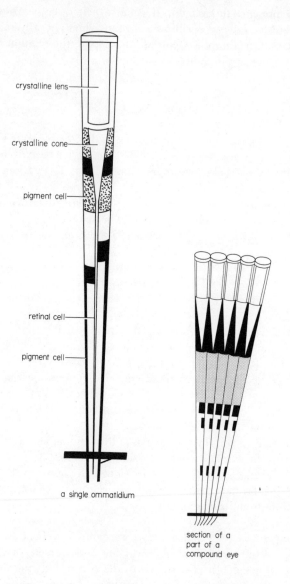

crystalline lens

crystalline cone

pigment cell

retinal cell

pigment cell

a single ommatidium

section of a
part of a
compound eye

Fig. 50 A single ommatidium and a section of part of a
compound eye.

insects are not merely light sensitive but can determine form and space with various degrees of visual acuity. They perceive movement and the spatial relationship of distant objects.

The total visual image received through a compound eye is composed of an aggregate of spots of light and darkness, comparable with a newspaper photograph.

Figuier estimated the number of facets in various compound eyes as follows:
Some beetles, 25 000 facets; dragon fly, 17 355; housefly, 4000; ants, 100–1000, varying with variety and sex.

COLOUR PERCEPTION THROUGH COMPOUND EYES

A tendency for any insect to visit flowers of a certain colour does not necessarily demonstrate the possession of colour vision. Some insects are able to discriminate between differences in the intensity of light reflected from various surfaces. However, it is known that insects may be stimulated by wavelengths between about 2500 Å and 7000 Å, and can often detect ultraviolet radiation invisible to human eyes. Surfaces reflecting such wavelengths may therefore appear brighter to the insect than those which do not do so. Nevertheless, in spite of these possibilities, it has been demonstrated that blue colour perception exists in bees, butterflies, two-winged flies (diptera) and in some beetles.

Bees recognise four colours, red, yellow, green and blue green. They can also perceive the plane of vibration of polarised light and this is made use of by foraging bees for direction finding. Certain insects commonly referred to as 'backswimmers', because they swim upside down, have only the posterior ommatidia fully sensitive to colour.

DORSAL OCELLI

Typically, these are three in number, arranged in a triangle, but the disposition may vary in different kinds of insects. In the Mayflies they are borne on the front of the head but in some insects the median ocellus is situated on the front of the head and the paired ocelli are located at the rear, between the compound eyes. These dorsal ocelli vary a great deal in the details of their construction.

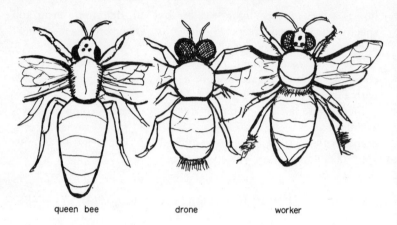

queen bee   drone   worker

Fig. 51   The Queen Bee, Drone, and Worker. Note comparative
size of the compound eyes, and the three ocelli on upper surface
of the head, arranged in a triangle.

THE CORNEA OF AN OCELLUS

The cornea in this case is the raised outside covering. The overlying cuticle is more transparent than elsewhere and usually it
becomes thickened to form a spherical lens. In the Mayflies the cornea
is arched but not thickened and the lens is made up from a mass of
polygonal cells underlying the corneagen layer.

The corneagen layer consists of colourless, transparent scales which
support the lens. In some insects the cells become grouped together
to form a vitreous body.

The retina of a dorsal ocellus is made up of sensory fibres which
constitute visual cells; each being connected by a nerve fibre. Two
or three cells become grouped together to form a retinula. The
retinula surrounds a longitudinal optic rod known as a rhabdon.

Pigment cells may exist in some occuli and play the part of an
iris.

FUNCTION

The purpose and function of the dorsal ocelli are not always clear.
Though the lens is capable of forming an image it would be focused
below the level of the retina and perception of form would therefore

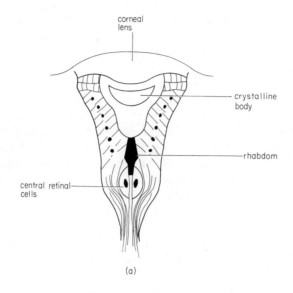

(a)

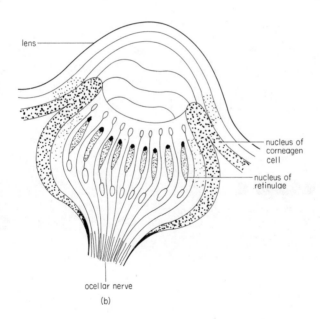

ocellar nerve

(b)

Fig. 52   Beetle ocelli. (a) Lateral and (b) dorsal.

be impossible. Blocking out the dorsal ocelli experimentally, slows down the rate at which the remaining visual processes operate and it is believed, therefore, that they may have an excitatory influence on other parts of the visual mechanism.

LATERAL OCELLI

These are the only eyes functioning in insect larvae. They are located on the sides of the head in the places finally occupied by the compound eyes. They are innervated by the optic lobes of the brain. Their number is variable, even in the same species of insect. In some instances a crystalline, refractive body may be developed below the corneal lens. Pigment granules may sometimes be absent.

Some insects possess lateral eyes with a distinctly ocilliform structure but which are not directly related either to compound eyes or to ocelli. In some kinds of lice there may be a single facet on either side of the head and in some of the wingless beetles, (Strepsiptera in particular,) about 50 facets may be found grouped together.

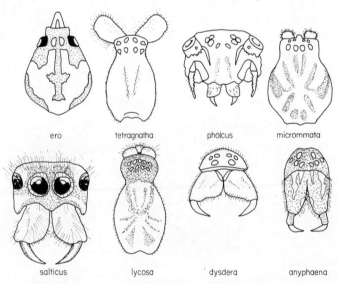

ero   tetragnatha   pholcus   micrommata

salticus   lycosa   dysdera   anyphaena

Fig. 53   Heads and faces showing the arrangement and number of ocelli; taken from a list of one hundred and fifty British species of spiders, and showing the different arrangement of ocelli.

SPIDERS

Although spiders build precise, geometrical webs, they do not *see* what they are doing. Their vision is not sufficiently good to enable them to control the procedure. The geometrical design must be associated with an instinctive need to arrange the filaments of the web in some direct relationship to their own limbs and body. Spiders

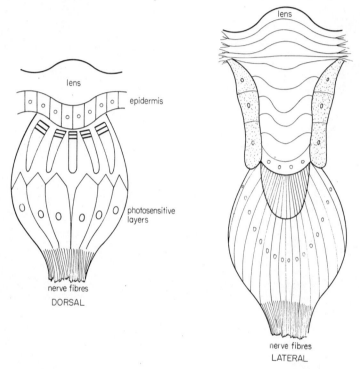

Fig. 54   Simple ocelli from a spider's eye.

have a collection of simple eyes, very crudely constructed, and some of these are placed in strange positions, high up on the head and not disposed to produce forward vision.

Four families have six and the remainder have eight eyes. W. S. Bristowe in his *World of Spiders*, considers that spiders *can* alter the focus of their eyes to suit given situations or requirements. It is unlikely that a spider can have any visual appreciation of the world more than six inches beyond its body. This applies to spiders that sit behind webs and depend upon vibration of strands to notify them of their catches.

The hunting spiders have better vision as they hunt and chase their prey and jump upon it but their eyes are simple and it is unlikely that the hunter can see many inches ahead.

CHAPTER 12
MISCELLANEOUS ANIMALS— NOTES ON SPECIAL PECULIARITIES

AMOEBA

As there is no brain there can be no reflexes. Light waves act directly on the cell causing movements within the *plasmosol*, the fluid part of the cytoplasm. This causes the amoeba to move through any fluid in which it exists.

ANTEATER

The eyes are set lower in the head than in any other mammal. The extreme in monocular vision.

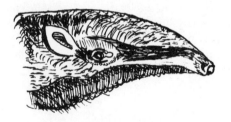

Fig. 55   Head of the Great Anteater.

APES

Vision similar to that of man.

BATS

Sight is elementary and not essential since the bat carries a highly efficient radar set based on supersonic hearing and echo perception. The body position in space is made evident and will prevent collision with any article thicker than a human hair.

BEAVERS

Have thickened corneae which enable them to see on land or under water.

BITTERN

This bird is able to raise its head with its long beak held high, and view the world behind its own throat. (See Fig. 34.) It has both central and temporal foveae.

BLEAK

It is universally believed by anglers that certain fish including bleak, roach, dace and salmon, prefer baits of certain colours according to the species, and refuse all others. With this belief in view they dye their maggots and select their feathers for fly fishing. Apart from this, presumably based on long experience, there is no scientific proof that fish behave in this way.

DOGFISH

The dogfish, sharks and rays are colour blind. All other fish can distinguish colours.

FLYING FOXES AND FRUIT BATS

Conical elevations on the choroid raise the retinal surface in places.

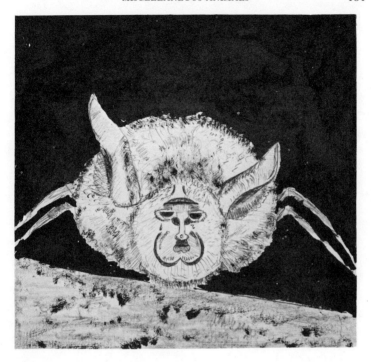

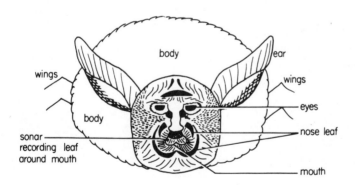

Fig. 56   The Greater Horshoe Bat. Note the minute eyes situated
on either side of the nose. The curved portion below the nose
and also surrounding it represents the nose-leaf, which directs
sound waves emitted through the nose during flight.

The rods above these are nearer to the lens. Sharp images are obtained by moving the head without making use of lens accommodation.

THE GUACHARO BIRD

This bird lives in dark caverns in Trinidad and Venezuela. Avoids walls while in flight by making clicking sounds and possibly high-frequency noises which are reflected back to the ears.

GURNARD

This fish spends its life deep down in complete darkness and possesses neither rods nor cones.

HERRING

This fish is provided with folds, or outgrowths of transparent skin which drop over the eyes.

KIWI

This New Zealand bird has the worst vision in the bird kingdom and sees little by night or day.

MOLE

An insectivorous animal with typical eyes; the smallest in existence; sometimes buried beneath the skin. See Fig. 57.

OPOSSUM

When the opossum closes its eyes the conjunctiva bulges out between the lids and resembles two large white tumours.

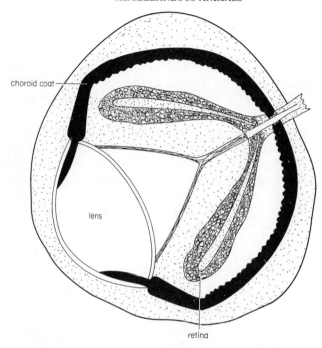

Fig. 57   The eye of the Mole. (From a photograph.)
   The eye is only 1 mm in diameter; it lay buried beneath the
skin. Some eyes are more superficial. The structure is that of an
embryonic eye and in the mole it does not advance further than
this stage of development. The lens is not clear because the
hyaloid artery has not been absorbed. The retina is funnel-
shaped and not in contact with the choroid coat. The mole
probably only sees enough to find entrance to its burrow after
wandering in search of worms.

OTTER

This animal has a ciliary muscle, but under water it contracts the
lens by means of the iris sphincter, just as the birds do. It sees
equally well on land and under water.

RODENTS

Rodents have a spherical lens which provides no power of accommodation and see equally badly in all parts of the retina. All have

lateral eye placement. The membrana nictitans has almost vanished in the small wild creatures such as mice, rats, shrews, hedgehogs, and moles.

Although in the true rodents the vision is so poor, they are able to see through the whole 360 degrees, but cannot see what goes on a few feet ahead, unless they tip the head and view with one eye at a time.

In rodents, as in bats, the retina occupies a much greater portion of the fundus than it does in most other mammals, which accounts for the wider range of vision. In some rodents and in lagomorphs (rabbit family) the two eyeballs may work independently, with regard to any movement they have.

Rodents seldom see a person if he, or she, makes no movement, but their eyes respond immediately to very slight movements.

Rabbits and hares, though not true rodents, can see what goes on behind them, even at full gallop.

THE SPECTRAL TARSIER

A tiny nocturnal lemur, resident in Borneo, owns the largest mammalian eyes in the world when compared with its body size.

The smallest eyes, on the same basis, are owned by the whale.

TROUT

The eye is supplied with blood from a 'false gill'. It is believed that it has the best chance of binocular vision among fishes of its kind.

VULTURES

Have the least high development among the flesh eaters. They depend for their food location upon the sense of smell.

WATER VOLES AND RATS

Keep their eyes closed when swimming below water.

WORMS

Earthworms work in the dark but need to come to the surface at intervals if only to get rid of their casts. They are safer below ground as they have no true eyes, only 'eyespots', which tell the worm the difference between light and darkness. They are grouped mainly at either end of the body with a few scattered over the remainder of the body surface.

Worms make use of their eyespots in the breeding season when half the body has to be exposed to light while the other half remains in the earth.

Some other worms, the planaria, have eyespots in the head end of the body so arranged that they can locate the direction from which the light originates. They then turn towards or away from the light according to their needs.

CRABS, LOBSTERS, SHRIMPS AND PRAWNS

All of these enjoy comparatively good vision in water, with some degree of colour appreciation.

A great many crabs, particularly the soft-shelled crabs and those which favour beaches and estuaries, appear to be able to see on land. Some of the latter will reach out their claws to grasp small objects moved slowly in front of their bodies. They do not appear to see objects behind their heads. A crab in a rock pool can see quite well for as long as the pool is lit by sunlight. In darkness, crabs are believed to rest unless something very attractive comes into reach. Some young crabs have eyes mounted on stalks like those of garden snails. It is believed that they see well enough but without great detail. It is probable that crabs and lobsters have a keen sense of taste and can locate food materials some distance away by flavours carried in the water.

The crayfish has eyes mounted on short stalks. The eyes are compound and constructed much on the lines of those of an insect. See Fig. 58.

Shrimps have compound eyes. If a torch is shone on the head-end of a shrimp at night, the eye reflects the light and appears as a pool of magenta. Their eyes adapt themselves to the existing intensity of light. By day the eyes show a dark central spot surrounded

F

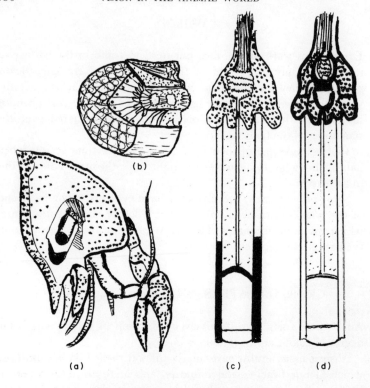

Fig. 58   Head of a crayfish, showing stalked eye.
(a)   Fore-end of the crayfish showing the stalked, tubular eye.
This is nevertheless a typical compound eye.
(b)   Shows the eye in section.
(c)   The body of the eye is made up of columns of ommatidia
(c) and (d).
      In (c) the pigment insulates the walls during exposure to
bright light.
      In (d) (for darkness) the pigment moves down out of the way.

by a yellow rim. The pigment has retreated to the depth of the eye.
By night the pigment travels to the outer circumference and surrounds each crystalline cone. This gives the eye its black appearance
and the retina becomes visible and provides the magenta reflection.
Shrimps and prawns appear to see well under water and are
immediately responsive to a finger held up over their pool.

They use their eyes also to vary their body colour so that it will
harmonise with that of their environment, for just so long as the light
remains sufficiently good to make colour contrasts recognisable.

INTRO FINAL.

Obedience
Cog Diss
Attribution   Attitudes
interpers. Attraction

SNAILS AND SLUGS

These actually see only a matter of inches but their power of smell can detect food six feet distant—or more. The snails have stalked eyes which can be adjusted. They also have pores in the skin, covered by a thin transparent film, curved to act as a lens, focusing light onto a sensitive floor. The stalked eye of the snail has a lens made up of stiff jelly, with an elementary retina.

OCTOPUSES AND SQUIDS

In the cephalopods—the octopuses, squids and cuttlefish—the eye loses its simplicity and becomes complex. The eyes are very similar to those of mammals.

In the Nautilus, (the Portuguese Man-of-War), which has an outer shell, there is only a 'pinhole camera', in which the light enters a minute hole in the skin and is focused onto photosensitive cells lying at the bottom of a pit. The difficulty in these cuticular eyes is that there is no definite brain capable of receiving and interpreting visual impressions.

In squids, cuttlefish and octopuses, we encounter the perfect eye; so much so that these creatures possess the best sight to be found in the invertebrates. The squid sees as well under water as any fish. It has no focusing mechanism but is purely automatic since the retina is able to cope with any focus within the animal's reach of vision. The rods and cones are so increased in length that the image can advance and recede throughout the focal radius of the animal's vision. Whether the brain is capable of translating the image is another matter.

OYSTERS AND LIMPETS

The eyes of the limpet are only little pits in the skin without a lens, with only a few retina cells and some pigment at the receiving end. The eye merely recognises light.

The eyes of the oyster are similar and the only reaction they induce is to close the shell when light appears. On the other hand the scallop, which moves about in the water by a system of pro-

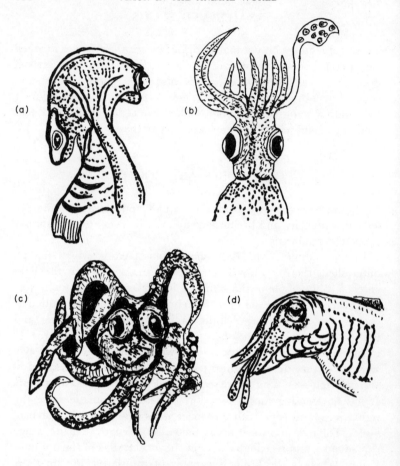

Fig. 59   (a) The head of a hammer-headed shark; (b) the head of a squid; (c) head of an octopus; (d) head of a cuttlefish.

pelling jets of water through the openings between its shells, has over a hundred eye spots arranged along the insides of the shells, near their edges. They merely register light which causes the scallop to close its shell and sink into darker surroundings.

Each of its eyespots boasts a lens and a retina connected to a branch of the optic nerve.

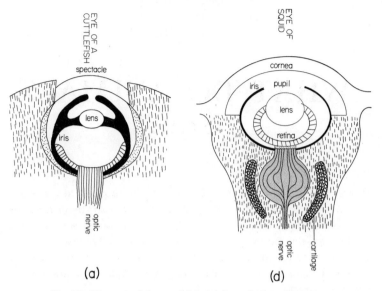

(a)   (d)

Fig. 60 The eye of the cuttlefish (a) is perfectly adjusted to underwater vision; since the focal length of the visual cells in the retina have been increased in length, they cater for all ranges of vision without any need for adjustment. The eye of the squid (b) follows on the same lines but is even more detailed.

CHAPTER 13

WHAT DO ANIMALS SEE?

Before we attempt to calculate how much animals actually see, we must make it clear that although we can determine the structure of each eye and how the eye functions, we are quite unable to determine how the animal actually interprets the image formed on the retina. From the animals' reactions to visual stimuli we can form our own conclusions, but these may not be entirely correct.

In previous chapters we have studied the eyes of a great many animals: their structure, how they deal with the matter of accommodation and how they have become adapted to different environments. Before proceeding further it may be fitting if we devote a little thought to a very important aspect of animal vision, and that is, What do animals really see? How capable are they of distinguishing detail in objects close to their eyes, and how far away from their eyes can they still recognise distant objects? How does their acuity of vision differ from our own and how much information can they acquire from the visual image they receive, and how do they react to it? In other words, how does the world appear to animal eyes? To do this we shall have to consider animals varying immensely in size, and shape, each with its own particular environment and its special needs. We shall also be compelled to determine how important vision is to any particular animal and what role the other senses play in the animal's life and its way of living.

The acuity of vision demanded in a falcon which hovers hundreds of feet above the earth's surface while it seeks a mouse among the foliage, is very much greater than that required by the spider which sits in the corner of its web awaiting a visitor. We must not forget, however, that the spider has actually built the web on a most intricate geometrical pattern without making a single mistake and without prior tuition. How great a part vision plays in this undertaking will be discussed later in this chapter.

Then we must include the shag which chases a fish under water, peering through a transparent window in its third eyelid and keeping ten feet away, until it makes its final rush in, to gather the fish and bring it to the surface in its beak before it endeavours to swallow it.

And what about the fish? How do fishes see under water and how much can they see through spectacles and a cornea? How does the refractive index of the latter compare with that of the medium in which the fish swims?

There are other creatures which live below water at times and on dry land at others. They include the aquatic mammals, such as the hippopotamus, which comes ashore by day but soaks in a mud bath by night, with turret eyes which can enable it on occasion to sleep with its eyes and nostrils above water level, while its body is submerged, and the frogs, which spend nearly as much time below water as they do above it, and which also possess the turrets which enable them to float just below water level, with the eyes taking in all other objects on the neighbouring surface.

Then again, the mussels, and the limpets which spend so much of their time exposed to the sun as it strikes the rock, only to become submerged some hours later, in a regular rhythm.

The lives of all these animals, what they see, and how much they need to see, must be entirely different. What is essential is that not only by vision, but by utilising a variety of senses, each of these individual creatures may be enabled to exist, reproduce its kind, and live a life normal to its nature.

The demands upon animal intellect, which include an interpretation of the visual image, are not so stringent as they are in our own species. They have no occasion to read small print, nor to study the intricate workings of a wrist watch. What they most need is to find a safe spot in which to live and recognise food, and determine how to secure it. Their other requirement is to reproduce their kind. In order to do this they need to be able to recognise a difference between the sexes before making closer contact. It may seem curious that dogs appear visually unable to distinguish the sex of their fellows, even when it is apparent to the human eye. They depend entirely upon the sense of smell and their ability to differentiate the respective odours is possible even, on occasion, at a distance.

Something which strikes one as being rather curious is that a few of the better developed animals such as the dogs, which possess good eyes, include a variety of types, each of which differs in the value it attaches to vision and the amount of co-operation it derives from other senses. Among the canines in domestication we encounter the gazehounds, comprising a number of breeds, each of which hunts entirely by vision; in addition to the hound group are the gundogs which depend entirely upon their sense of smell, even when the creature they are hunting eventually comes into full view.

Shooting men are quite familiar with the spaniel or retriever seeking a 'runner', a bird, or a rabbit which is wounded but able to run, that sticks so closely to the scent that it ends up by tumbling over the game before it realises that it is directly in its path, even when it was actually in full view if the dog had made use of its eyes. Hounds, hunting in a pack, make use of peripheral vision to keep in touch with the other members, but a pack of foxhounds will hunt with scent breast-high and yet make no extra effort to increase their pace, apparently quite oblivious to the fact that a tired fox is just ahead and in full view if they care to look straight ahead. The terrier that catches rats, will find whether the latter are at home by means of its nose, but the moment the rat comes into the open the scent of smell is immediately discarded and vision comes into full use. If, however, the rat reaches fresh cover still unharmed, the terrier will revert to scent, until it is once more unearthed and in the open, when vision again takes over. These variations appear to exist, not because the sense of smell, or that of vision, is in any way lacking, but because the particular variety of dog has a preference for one or other of the senses.

One is at a loss to know whether animals see things in the same way as we, ourselves, do, or even how much they can learn from a visual image which is as perfect as it can be. Animals seldom gather anything from looking at a large or even a life-size picture of a person or another animal, and it is only the exceptional dog or cat in the home that can recognise another dog or cat on a television screen for what it is.

Even when a dog is barking loudly and in full view on the screen, it is only rarely that a dog by one's fireside will take any notice. If, by any chance, it is impressed by the barking, it rarely associates it with anything evident on the screen. It must be remembered though that uneducated people are almost as incapable of interpreting a picture as the dog is when a screen picture is concerned.

Many African natives of today given a black and white drawing or print depicting everyday objects, will turn the picture upside down and view it from every angle without realising what it represents.

Only occasionally does a dog recognise a life-size painting of one of its kind. The late Professor McCunn of the Royal Veterinary College, kept a painting of a Pekinese on the wall of his consulting room. Out of all the patients that passed through the room, only one recognised the painting. This dog was also a Pekinese and every time it was brought to see the professor, the picture had to be removed from the wall, otherwise the visiting Peke became frantic.

In my own consulting room I had a lifesized painting of one of my own Fox terriers standing in the empty fireplace as a screen. It was not unusual for a visiting dog to stand spellbound before the screen, then run up to it and cock a leg on it. Whether this indicated a correct interpretation of a visual image or whether the picture had acquired an inviting odour, I could never ascertain. It is to be presumed that the retinal image presented to a bird with a pecten, or to a horse with a ramp retina, is not unlike that which falls upon the human retina but as has been remarked elsewhere in this book, the brain itself has to be educated before it can translate the message into a brain picture. The building-up of the latter is very involved and associated with the amount of nerve decussation present in the optic chiasma. Even our own eyes often provide us with images we do not understand. The child in infant school is presented with such undecipherable images many times in a day but the salient features are explained and in many instances the child is allowed to play with an unusual object or handle it so as to develop an association between vision and touch. Animals have to learn the hard way but although the feeding bowl may mean nothing to the puppy that has recently opened its eyes, its sense of smell soon convinces it that the bowl deserves further attention and the lesson is learned, and the recollection persists throughout life.

The Primates, in the same way as the Pugs and the Pekinese, possess frontal vision and this undoubtedly goes a long way towards presenting a picture discernable in three dimensions; though which animals possess true stereoscopic vision is never certain, although a study of the optic chiasma in the particular species may once more assist in coming to a decision.

There is one virtue in binocular vision when applied to the beasts of the field. This is that animals possessing it can usually see all around them at once and even observe what goes on behind them.

A horse grazing from the ground can see in every direction without lifting the head, particularly because at whatever position the head may assume, the pupils of the eyes are carried horizontally and centrally.

Birds recognise their mates by the colouring of their feathers but in addition, they study behaviour and the dancing and posturing which may be associated with courtship, in each sex. When the female bower-bird watches another bird of her kind building a maypole nest, (resembling a fourposter bed lined with coloured shells and silver paper), her visual images assure her that the bird, so hard at work, is a male, and on offer, unless she can observe another little female standing shyly by. The toothbill does not build a bower but makes a clearing on the ground and decorates it with coloured leaves.

A fish's eye-view is quite different from that of a bird although it may include objects derived from the land on the banks of a river or lake. Even if some fishes have a certain amount of colour vision, it can be put to practical use only when the light rays are able to penetrate the water to some depth. In these favourable circumstances a fish can see very well, as it has a good retina and a cornea which is adapted to underwater vision.

In aquatic animals such as seals and whales, the surface of the eye is flattened, and whales probably see nothing when their heads are out of the water. The seal does very well when it allows the contracted slit pupil to cross the normal line of astigmatism present in every seal's eye, thus producing a perfect replica of the pinhole camera, an arrangement which provides good vision without the necessity of focusing.

Reverting to the amount of vision available to a fish underwater, let us find out how much it can see of what goes on in the world around it. People who dive with the aid of goggles and an aqualung may be able to provide first-hand information. In a narrow river or in a pond, a fish can often see above the surface as well as below it. Its range of vision includes a dome above its head extending into the atmosphere above water. It can look up towards the sky and see objects in the air, and according to its depth or its nearness to the surface it can see objects on the bank (if the bank is close by) at a range permitted, supposing a line from the fish's eye met the water level at an angle of forty five degrees. The deeper the fish lies the greater is the circle of vision but the less is the illumination. If the fish were swimming only a few feet below the surface its view of the surroundings above water would be excellent.

When a fish directs its eyes upwards at an oblique angle with the surface of the water, it can no longer see through the surface but sees a reflection of objects resting on the sea bed reflected on the under surface of the water, which acts like a mirror, as well as a reflection of the sea bed within the circle. The apparent distance between the reflection and the fish will depend upon the angle from

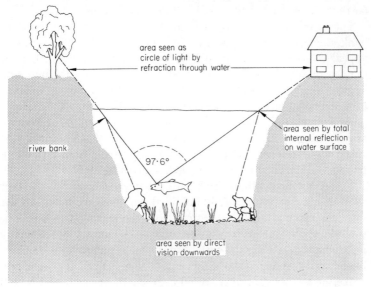

area seen as circle of light by refraction through water

area seen by total internal reflection on water surface

river bank

97·6°

area seen by direct vision downwards

Fig. 61   Vision of fish underwater.

which the reflections are viewed. The light from above the water will pass through the sea water to the sea bed from which some light will be reflected back. If this reflected light strikes the surface at an angle less than ninety degrees it will not pass through the surface but will be reflected back again. (Internal reflection.)

A fish, looking up at the water surface at such an angle, will not see *through* the surface but will see a reflected image of part of the sea bed, outside the circle of vision which it has of the world above the water; it will see this because of refraction of light through the surface when it looks up to the surface at a lesser angle.

According to the depth at which the fish lies, the surface reflection will convey a picture of all solid objects between the centre of the circle and a restricted circle of light above the water. If the surface of the water is calm and smooth, it will reflect and permit the fish to view objects which lie *above* water level. The clearness of the picture will depend upon the smoothness of the surface, and the angle at which the rays of sunlight impinge upon the water surface, as well as upon whether the water is murky or clear. Anglers will realise that all these factors decide whether the fish he wishes to catch can see his intention or be oblivious to his presence. The illustration (Fig. 61) will explain more clearly how much and how far the fish sees under different conditions or lighting.

The nearer the solid object is to the edge of the pond or river bank, the larger it will appear in the reflection, although it will still appear relatively small. An angler, seated on the bank will look to the fish under water like a tiny doll at the window edge but if he decides to stand up suddenly and peer into the water he will immediately assume a great size and appear to be floating in space or hanging over the surface of the window, which is sufficient to drive any self-respecting fish a mile upstream; all of which makes it surprising that a fisherman casting a fly repeatedly from a standing position on the river bank, ever catches anything at all.

Whatever the depth, in fresh water (not seawater) and wherever the fish may be lying, the illuminated window, overhead, always subtends an angle of 97·6 degrees from the eyes of the fish. The position of the sun at any given time determines the amount of light which penetrates the surface of the lake, providing the surface of the water is reasonably calm at the time. When the light rays strike the water at an angle of 60 degrees, 18 per cent will be lost through reflection and 72 per cent will penetrate the water. If the rays strike the surface at an angle of 10 degrees, 72 per cent is lost through the reflection and 18 per cent will penetrate the surface.

G. L. Walls, in *The Vertebrate Eye*, stated that off Plymouth (Devon), 90 per cent of white light was extinguished at 8–9 metres depth and 99 per cent at 35 metres. In the clearest waters utter darkness exists at 535 metres. In dirty harbours, light only penetrates a few metres. Ultraviolet light is almost totally absorbed in the first few millimetres of water, though traces reached 1000 metres and were recorded on a photographic plate after an exposure of 80 minutes. A goldfish sees more of the outside world and of its human protectors if it is kept in a jar with flat sides than if kept in a round bowl in which light refraction may produce some strange effects from the optical standpoint. Whether it is kinder to the fish to provide a flat bowl or a round one may require consideration according to circumstance.

Fish are extremely sensitive to vibration, which is transmitted through the water from the earth. The monks used to call fish to feed by ringing a bell. Hob-nailed boots on a river bank will scare fish and so will sudden movements from a figure which has previously been sitting. Even knocking out a pipe on a stone will act similarly.

It is debateable whether a book dealing with vision is entitled to discuss 'second sight', but we are justified in pointing out that during the course of evolution, dogs (which we will choose as an example since most people have enjoyed some degree of acquaintance with them), have retained certain senses and sensitivities which we humans have lost. Apart from their uncanny sense of smell, which we have also lost, dogs possess what has been termed a sixth sense which enables at least a few of them, on occasion, to find their way across hundreds of miles of country while others cannot find their own front gate if inadvertently they become lost during a short walk. This is no place to recount dog stories but the following, vouched for by Emeritus Professor H. G. Lamont of Belfast University, himself a veterinary surgeon, is worthy of mention if only on account of the amount of vision needed to ensure its success. I have recorded this story previously in *The Mind of the Dog*.

Dinah, was a Red Setter bitch, belonging to the Professor's mother. She was sent by train from Cookstown in Northern Ireland, to Lurgan, a matter of 25 miles. Shortly after her arrival she whelped five puppies, then promptly disappeared from her new home, puppies and all. She had previously never been outside Cookstown. Ten days later she was found asleep in her old bed at Cookstown with the five puppies, all alive and well, tucked in beside her. Her feet were raw and bleeding and she was dreadfully emaciated.

Obviously she had travelled on foot and must have transported the five puppies in relays over short distances, so how many times she actually covered the mileage is unknown. On her journey back to Cookstown she swam, complete with her family, the River Blackwater at Maghery Ferry, where it is over 80 yards wide and very deep, a number of times in each direction, carrying one puppy at a time and leaving some of her family on opposite shores until she had completed their transport.

In due course Dinah recovered, reared all her puppies and remained a resident in Cookstown for the remainder of her days.

It must again be emphasised that the ability to *see* one's way across miles of unknown country is not innate in every dog, any more than the ability to divine water is present in every person. The ability appears to be linked with maturity, as puppies up to twelve months old remain lost with unfailing regularity. Probably it takes time for 'home' to make its imprint on the mind.

Experiments made on the ability of lost dogs to find their way home through unknown territory have shown that a dog first wanders around the immediate locality, quite vaguely, for about half an hour. It then seems to derive inspiration regarding the correct direction and makes off with evident purpose. After a short while the inspiration fails and the dog is again lost. This may happen many times on a long journey but each time after a spell of vague wandering, inspiration appears to return and the dog travels a few more miles on the correct course. The dog rarely travels in a circle. Each burst of progress appears always to be in the right direction.

The everyday flights of homing pigeons are equally amazing and nobody has offered any explanation other than the employment of a superior grade of vision, even if this is not altogether convincing. Fanciers look in their birds' eyes for what they term 'eye-sign', a peculiar film-like circle in the iris immediately surrounding the pupil. Whether this means anything or nothing is not certain. It could be associated with pecten development, or with the super-development of a fovea—more probably neither. No certain reason has yet been brought forward to explain adequately how birds migrate across oceans to a definite location. All that is known is that at great heights they close the membrana nictitans and 'fly blind'.

We know more about the dog than about most animals as man and dog have lived together for probably a million years and must by now have formed pretty definite ideas concerning each other's behaviour. When we consider the matter of canine vision we have to take into consideration the part played by other senses. We have already discussed the difference between the gazehounds and the scent hounds and drawn attention to the useful part the dog's nose plays in the matter of sex detection. Police dogs nowadays have been trained to ferret out clothing and even a handkerchief owned by suspected criminals, and to find drugs concealed in the most unlikely situations; something which they could never achieve by vision. It has been shown that a dog can detect a scent only just recognisable by a human nose, after it has been diluted 150 times.

No wonder when we take our dog for a country walk, it is far more interested in sniffing the hedges than in admiring the scenery. And yet, whenever anything moves, whether it be a bird, a cat or a rabbit, the dog's attention is immediately diverted to the moving object and for a brief moment all smells are forgotten.

Birds are also remarkably quick at detecting movement and it is therefore the more surprising that although they pay no attention to leaves and branches moving in the breeze, or during a storm, they immediately observe the movement of a living person or animal in the midst of such an environment.

The ability of insects to fly from considerable distances towards the smell from possible food is only too well-known. One might imagine that a wasp or a bluebottle would employ the sense of smell to bring it into touch with the article of food and that once in its vicinity it would make use of vision. But this does not appear to be the case. A wasp flies from one end of a beach to the other the moment some happy picnicker opens a tin of pears, but once in close proximity, the concentration of odour in the air seems to puzzle the wasp as to its precise point of origin. One would think that its compound eyes would immediately observe the open tin and that the mission would be completed but this does not happen and the wasp is still undecided whether the food lies in someone's tea cup, or on the fingers of the lady who opened the tin of pears. The reason for this is that the wasp is susceptible to a highly diluted odour but its senses become overwhelmed when the odour is highly concentrated, and its acuity of vision is insufficient to enable it to distinguish the source from a number of possible sources.

We will deal further with insects in flight a little later. Among other animals, one of the most interesting, owing to its power to survive and multiply, is the common house mouse. Like many of the other rodents, the mouse has rather poor vision but it has a remarkable ability to detect both ground vibration and movement, which it uses as its main protection against possible enemies. Its range of vision, using its spherical lens, is very limited when compared with that of man, its principal enemy. But the mouse is also endowed with very keen hearing and can appreciate sound waves outside the human appreciation and can probably communicate with its fellows in tones we do not hear. Moreover, a mouse hidden on the ground beneath a dock leaf, can hear the ultrasonic fluttering of the wings of the hawk hovering fifty yards overhead and knows enough to 'freeze' and remain quite motionless until the hawk has sought fields and pastures new. But the mouse is not so lucky when it comes out at night, seeking the advantage of darkness, for the owls are about. Although the mouse is unaware of the fact, its body is emitting infra-red rays which *we* would not be able to see but which would be quite apparent to the eyes of the owl.

The spider, cunningly concealed in the corner of its web, may not be able to see the gnat which has become entangled in its meshes, but it is extremely susceptible to vibration. Not only can it detect by this means the presence of the insect but it can estimate its size and in exactly which part of the web it is being held. The spider will then streak across the web to the correct spot, feel the insect with its palps and administer the fatal dose of poison, possibly without ever 'seeing' the victim. The spider would only recognise the lady who dusts away its web as an indistinct blob, even if it observed her presence at all, but it would register all the sounds and vibrations attendant upon her efforts to destroy it, and when the pace became too hot it would 'freeze', and pretend to be dead.

A spider, sitting in the centre of a web in the garden, will allow you to approach within a foot of it providing your movements are slow. It ignores a slight breeze but if you blow very gently on a corner of the web and set it into sudden vibration, the spider will disappear immediately into its 'parlour', sited at one corner of its web. Spiders have simple eyes on top of the head and different varieties have definite arrangements of more eyes on the body, chiefly on the under surface, often four or five on one spider. None of these appear to be very efficient but no doubt they have their uses.

There are some other factors which play a part in certain kinds of animals and exert a marked influence upon what they can or cannot see. One of these is the question of the animal's horizon, or in other words, how close are the eyes to the ground? Another factor which is of importance, particularly so far as distant vision is concerned, is the type and shape of the animal's retina.

First, let us consider the position of the animals in relation to the ground, particularly those which live mainly on the earth's surface, or in the air, or swim in water. The distance between the horizon and the eyes, how far the eyes lie above ground level, and the ability of the animal to recognise distant objects, are all matters to be taken into account.

The dog has a relatively good vision over a distance. A greyhound, for example, can see a moving rabbit, but not necessarily a still one, at a distance of a hundred yards, and possibly further if the light is particularly good. But let us now compare the greyhound with a Pekinese, which has large, open eyes, placed almost fully frontally, and only about six inches above ground level.

If the little dog is taken for a walk running along beside its owner on a short lead, through a busy city, making use of the pavements, the possible range of vision allotted to the dog cannot exceed a matter of twelve feet even supposing it could see over such a distance without marked obstruction to its gaze.

But a Pekinese would not be likely to see any great distance at all, because cavorting around its head and body would be a forest of human legs and feet. Its chief attention will be directed towards manoeuvring between these to avoid being trodden underfoot. Depending as it normally would upon its nose rather than its eyes in such circumstances, it finds itself defeated by a heterogeneous assortment of strange scents, combined with that of thousands of human bodies. A very trying situation for a proud little descendant of celestial origin, used to the privacy of the Palace.

If we take a greyhound into a five acre field and give it freedom, the dog will canter around with its head moving from side to side and up-and-down, in order that it may transfer the direction of its vision to various parts of the field before any likely quarry is able to make a getaway, unchallenged. Every now and then it will take short jumps up into the air in order to obtain a longer range of view. or it may take advantage of any high ground or hillock from which it may see farther afield.

Another creature, a spider for example, would be at no greater advantage if transported onto a hillock in the middle of a grass field than would the greyhound, if it were shut in a sitting room corner, keeping watch over a web. Animals are constructed for particular purposes and their eyes are designed for one particular need. Very few sets of visual apparatus could be made interchangeable.

Almost every mobile animal experiences a desire to see more of what goes on in its vicinity than its opportunities naturally permit. A cat climbs a tree to see further afield. A stoat or a ferret will bounce up and down on the grass in a pasture with the idea that some unfortunate rabbit may be squatting unobserved.

Birds of prey, notably the hawks and the eagles, possess amazingly good distance vision, far superior to that of man, and in addition, they own flexible necks which permit their heads to turn rapidly in any direction. Possessing, as every member of the hawk family does, an excellent retina, with double foveae and binocular, stereo-scopic vision, it is favoured with the best long distance sight in the animal kingdom.

In birds such as the gannets and the shags, we find good distance vision and an ability to detect the presence of shoals of fish by changes in the tone or colouring of the surface water. A gannet can visualise a shoal five hundred feet below it; will close its third eyelids to protect its eyes, then fall blindly with its beak outstretched ready to impale any fish in its downward dive through the water. On the other hand, a falcon will dive one thousand feet down to pick up a roving mouse with eyes open in order that it may watch the movements of the mouse and arrive at the right spot at the right fraction of a second.

In all birds which search the ground beneath them while in flight, as well, perhaps, as fishes which patrol beneath the surface, the distance at which the eye functions most successfully may bear a definite relationship to the distance through the eyeball from front to back. In individual eyes this may imply that the distance between cornea and lens is correspondingly reduced and when this happens and the eye is provided with a highly contractile pupil, the need for further measures towards accommodation may be negligible, although such an arrangement will be less reliable when objects close at hand require to be examined in detail.

Members of the hawks and eagles, birds which have superlative vision, have eyes short from front to back but provided also with especially effective means of accommodation and with high grade cones packed within the retina, a million to each square millimetre. Such eyes are ideally suited to birds which fly high in the sky and yet need to keep a close watch upon small creatures on the ground surface. Not only do birds of prey have to locate these but they need to keep them constantly in focus during the whole of their lightning-like descent to earth. The owls on the other hand, birds which hunt mainly by night but occasionally during the hours of daylight, need an entirely different eye, adaptable to needs similar to those of the hawks, but with one outstanding difference; the favourite height of a prowling owl, from the ground, is in the region of twenty-five feet.

As we noted in an earlier chapter the ability of an owl to see its prey from a moderate height is enhanced by the frontal position of its eyes and the very remarkable ability of the owl to swivel the head into any position; upside down or back to front, being within its facile range. It has therefore all the advantages of binocular vision with stereoscopic ability and a mechanism akin to a telescope mounted on a swivelling tripod.

Another feature which influences visual ability in a great many animals of various kinds is the degree of convexity of the cornea, and the amount of proptosis present, which means to say the amount of cornea visible between the upper and lower eyelids. The cornea combines with the lens to form a compound lens, the power of which will depend to some extent on the convexity of the cornea as well as upon the shape of the lens. One must also take into consideration the anterior chamber of the eye, filled with the aqueous humour; which together act in the same way as a simple lens situated in front of the iris, with the other portion of the compound lens lying behind it. The different effect upon the diopter count of an eye provided with a convex cornea, as in a hawk, or a flat cornea, as in a fish, can be readily realised, particularly when one remembers that the hawk has a biconvex lens whilst the fish has a round one. This is without taking into consideration the difference in the refractive ratios of air and water. A cod with a hawk's eye, even if the cornea were flattened with a protective spectacle, would be at a considerable disadvantage; but no greater than the hawk that exchanged eyes with a cod. In either of these so much must also depend upon the degree of accommodation available. A lens is of no optical value unless it can be brought into focus. It is always possible that when a cornea protrudes unduly from between the eyelids and when it is markedly convex, distant vision may be at a disadvantage.

In man this can be overcome by bifocal lenses, which cannot be used in other animals; at least not by those living in the wild.

Apropos of this, I myself owned a Cairn terrier which had both lenses removed on account of cataract and thereafter went its walks wearing a pair of 10 diopter lenses fitted into leather goggles. Thus equipped, it had no difficulty in following and avoiding even small obstacles.

It is remarkable that the largest animals in existence at present, such as the elephant, the whale and the hippopotamus have relatively the smallest eyes among living creatures. It is possible that the possession of sufficient size and strength makes such animals formidable and less in need of an 'escape reaction'. It is doubtful whether the whale can see anything when its eyes are above water level and the stories we read about whales chasing and turning over boats sent out to capture them may in most cases have been based on ignorance of the facts, or on pure coincidence.

The elephant has good close-up vision but its eyes do not see objects clearly at any great distance, which is fortunate for people who have unwittingly approached, rather too closely, elephants in African countries without being aware of their presence. An elephant depends largely upon ground vibration to detect the approach of other animals. It has good hearing but its ear flaps do not always assist the process of hearing.

The horse with its larger eye and ramp retina, has far better distant vision especially when it can keep the head raised to avoid interference to vision by its large foreface. It has also a wide range of vision using one eye at a time, as well as binocular vision, straight ahead, to include distant objects. This is why certain race horses run better in blinkers, which prevent them becoming preoccupied with happenings other than winning races.

Horses also have an excellent view of the land in front, behind and all around them when their heads are held down while they are grazing. They then make use of binocular and monocular vision at will and can see behind their bodies by monocular vision. The eyes of horses, as of most ungulates, are held horizontally, whatever the position of the head.

In the Primates, men and the apes, the retina is almost circular but in most other animals it is asymmetrical and arranged usually in such a way as to provide the view, or outlook, best suited to the needs of the particular species. In most herbivorous animals the retina is usually wider in the vertical than in the transverse direction so that it provides a view of what goes on above the head and around the feet, rather than what goes on at either side. An exception seems to be in the domestic cow which has good lateral vision, possibly associated with a ramp retina, which enables it to see its own calf while it sucks. This peculiarity is more apparent in some of the dairy breeds than in the beef breeds and may be a genetic factor introduced by selective breeding.

In the carnivorous animal, the retina is usually wider on the temporal than on the nasal side, as opposed to that in the herbivora.

This enables the animal, when hunting, to see better in a forward direction and keep the hunted creature in view. The retinal image, after passing through the compound lens of the eye, becomes completely reversed. In addition, objects on the right hand side of the field of vision appear on the left hand side of the retina, and vice versa. We, and other animals, are not conscious of this because the brain corrects the impression and permits objects to be observed in their normal position.

A man, a mile away, appears on the retina of a horse as an image 1/880 of an inch in height. In the human eye the picture of a man at the same distance would measure 1/500 of an inch in height; equal to the size of a red corpuscle in the blood. In the retina of a horse a six foot man standing at a distance of ten yards, would occupy one fifth of an inch, while in the eye of a man, it would be a little over one eighth of an inch.

But, in point of fact, the size of that image is not the all-important factor, what really matters is how much of the visual impression the animal can convert into a mental image that it can understand.

The estimation of distance is more or less a matter of education and it is believed that in other animals the ability to make such an estimate is not well developed. It is obvious that show-jumping horses, are able to estimate the distance between jumps, somewhat crowded together in an indoor jumping exhibition, but not so well in open country where the jumps are scattered at irregular intervals. The rider may help but a good rider does not necessarily make a good horse. Show jumpers quickly learn when the distance to a jump is too great or too little to be exactly right for the ensuing take-off, they are able, by changing the rhythm of the leading fore-leg to alter the distance by half a horse's length which usually puts the matter in order.

Man is apt to determine the distance of an object from his eyes by comparing his position in space with that of some other object, the distance of which from his eyes, is already known. But even keen rifle shots are unable to judge distance sufficiently well to decide whether the sights should be set for 300 or 400 yards, which is why each competitor on an open range carries a rangefinder. If a dozen farm labourers were asked to estimate the distance from a rick of hay to the steeple of the village church, there would be twelve different answers and the variation between the farthest and the shortest estimation would be remarkable.

It would be of minor importance to a swallow sitting on a telegraph wire whether the destination in its view were two miles distant, or four miles. Its flight is fast and sure and its time is its own.

Animals which are hunted over the ground are seldom tall enough to see long distances, even if they had the ability, and they sense the approach of possible enemies by earth vibration and by smell. A stag can detect the approach of a man two hundred yards away if the wind is blowing towards itself. Birds have excellent distance vision and the advantage of observation from a height.

Anyone who is in the habit of walking in open spaces with a dog will possibly have noticed that when a report of a gun is heard, the dog will without hesitation turn its head in the right direction, that from which the sound originated. We ourselves are usually content to say that it came from some distance away without any suggestion as to the direction from which the report came. Unless the gun were fired within a distance of a hundred yards, and the man behind it were visible, any opinion would be based on guesswork. Hearing is only one of the series of senses and not the most important to mankind, although to a carnivorous animal it has greater value.

Experimentally, it has been shown that a dog shut in a dark box and lowered below the surface of the earth where it can see nothing of its surroundings, can detect the direction of a handbell or electric bell rung at any point up to 25 yards surrounding the buried box. It has been stated that other animals including deer and pigs, have the same ability for the direction sounding of extraneous noises but they do not equal the powers of a Rhesus monkey owned by me and which, blindfolded, and seated in a closed room, could announce loudly the approach of one particular car proceeding along a busy main street in company with a great variety of cars travelling in both directions, fifty yards before it reached the building. This monkey, incidentally, was an exponent in keeping with many of his kind, of the stenopaic pupil. He would catch a fly or a beetle, almost completely close the pupils of his eyes, hold the insect about three inches from his nose and with fingers and thumb dismember it one limb at a time: not a very pleasant thought but a wonderful tribute to visual capability.

We have already discussed the susceptibility of all animals from spiders to apes to the observation of movement and their ability to attract attention. So much so that thousands of greyhounds chase a moving object they can never catch and hundreds of thousands of excited humans watch their movement with rapt enthusiasm!

Now we will look into a rather different aspect of movement recognition.

PARALLAX

As we move our heads slowly from side to side keeping our eyes open and active, we may observe that fixed objects close to us move across the retina in a direction *opposite* to that in which the head is moving.

The farther away from the eyes any fixed object is, the more slowly it moves across the field of vision.

An object a considerable distance away may appear hardly to move at all and at great distances an object may appear to move in the same direction as the head.

It is this ability to compare distance with eye movement that enables a man, blind in one eye, to find his way about without colliding with objects such as doorways, or lamp posts or falling over the chairs in his sitting room. In the case of human beings the loss of an eye can be overcome to some extent by training and experience. We may therefore conclude that an animal with monocular vision such as a rabbit or a squirrel, may not suffer any great disadvantage, especially as such animals can see not only in front of their bodies but also behind.

It may be imagined, on the grounds that what one has never had one never misses, that animals born with monocular vision and registering two separate images may, as they grow up, develop other ways of measuring distance and judging the solidity of masses. At any rate, they have the satisfaction of enjoying a much wider range of vision, as each eye is covering a separate area. It is possible that in such cases the mental processes may be adapted to the situation, either genetically or through experience.

MOVEMENT IN INSECTS

Insects that possess compound and very large eyes see over an extensive area while in flight, since the eyes are arranged with the ommatidia facing in all directions to provide wide-angled vision.

It is unlikely that the compound eye can see objects far ahead with great clarity and much depends upon how capable the brain behind these eyes is of interpreting hundreds of little pictures, all slightly different, into one complete jigsaw. There is undoubtedly a keen ability to appreciate light and movement.

The natural instinct of an insect imprisoned in a room is to return to the wide open spaces and as these are representative of light and space, the bluebottle, bee or wasp and the butterfly, all make for light and freedom. That they should mistake a clear glass window pane for the road to freedom, or even worse, the light bulb, is unfortunate but an insect, like some of the higher animals, is open to error. The insect's reaction to stimuli were instituted many centuries before the invention of either glass or electricity.

The interesting point is that if we try to drive the insect out of the open window it will escape all kinds of obstacles, perhaps because like the bat, it produces some form of high frequency sound, possibly a form of wing hum, which changes in tone when the insect is approaching a solid obstacle. Whatever the reason it is rather surprising that a pane of glass does not give a warning. It is probable that it does so, but the instinct to escape into the open may be overwhelming.

Many flying insects, houseflies for instance, do not emit a hum that we can hear, but it seems likely that some dogs are conscious of sounds far higher in pitch than anything our ears will register and are able to distinguish between the sounds of bees, wasps, bluebottles and mosquitoes.

One of my own terriers spends the summer catching wasps in her mouth, but ignores every other flying insect even when they are all available.

It is possible that fast-flying insects, especially those that enter buildings, depend as much upon echo response as upon vision. But the recognition of the echo response demands more investigation and unless it is an appreciation of vibration it seems rather illogical to attribute its recognition to hearing, when insects are notoriously deaf.

If a fly is resting in the sugar bowl you can shout at it from across the table and it will not budge. But make a sudden movement or tap the table and the fly will be up and away, having recognised the vibration, of course, when hearing failed.

Insects which suck blood do not select their victims by sight or smell, but by what is known as 'thermometric evaluation'. A female mosquito, needing a feed of blood, will be guided to a likely person by recognition of warmth, even a fraction of a degree, emanating from a human body. Butterflies have a sense of smell but they also see objects fairly clearly up to a distance of four feet and they can detect movement at six feet. Their caterpillars have sets of light-sensitive, simple eyes, incapable of 'vision' for much more than a range of an inch. Similar eyes are encountered around the circumference of jelly fishes.

The purpose of such eyes, in caterpillars at least, is not so much to attract them to the source of light but to get away from it. It is as though the influence of light on the eye spots causes discomfort which induces the caterpillars to retreat *underneath* leaves, where they are less likely to be found by birds, although it is more probable that their retreat is merely a reflex response to the presence of light.

The fleas which live on diurnal animals have large eyes, but some fleas are without apparent eyes. Those that live mainly on hedgehogs and other nocturnal animals, are frequently blind.

The ants have both simple and compound eyes. It seems apparent from the activities of ants that they possess some degree of vision from their compound eyes. It has been suggested that ants may be able to see, at the infra-red end of the spectrum, colours denied to our vision. Bettles have eyes, but as they favour darkness and many like to bury themselves, it is unlikely they function in any marked degree. Their sense of touch is exaggerated and they are most happy when they can enter crevices, the boundaries of which make contact with a large portion of their body surface.

How much bees, wasps and other flying insects see while in the air has raised some controversy from time to time.

BIBLIOGRAPHY

Bristowe, W. S., *The World of Spiders*.

Chapman Pincher, *A Study of Fishes*.

Davis, G. G., *Applied Anatomy*.

Davson, Hugh, *Physiology of the Eye*.

Figuier, Louis, *The Insect World*.

Henderson, Thomson, *Principles of Ophthalmology*.

Hogan, Alvardo and Waddel, *Histology of the Human Eye*.

Imms, A. D., *General Textbook of Entomology*.

Mackean, D. C., *Introduction to Biology*.

Matthew and Knight, *Senses of Animals*.

Nicholas, E. and Gray, H., *Veterinary and Comparative Anatomy*.

Prince, J. H., *Comparative Anatomy of the Eye*.

Smith, F., *Veterinary Physiology*.

Smythe, R. H., *The Mind of the Dog; Veterinary Ophthalmology* (Second
Edition); *Haunts and Habits of Fishes; The Mind of the Horse*.

Stephenson, E. M. and Stewart, C., *Animal Camouflage*.

Walls, G. L., *The Vertebrate Eye*.

Wehner, R., *Visual System of Arthropods*.

INDEX

Accommodation, 24, 35, 38, 47, 65–71, 78, 82, 87–90, 95, 118
Albino, 47, 49
Adder, 114
Alligator, 19, 105, 116, 117
Amoeba, 129
Amphibians, 8, 83
Analeps, 107
Angle of vision, 49, 71, 72
Ants, 125, 159
Anteater, 129
Anglers' baits, 28
Antennae, 12
Apes, 27, 129
Aquatic animals, 114–118
Arctic fox, 64, 65
Arythmic animals, 28
Ass, 90
Astigmatism, 83, 95

Baits, 27, 28
Baleen whales, 94
Bats, 21, 130
Bat radar, 21
Bear, 18
Beaver, 130
Bees, colour perception in, 28, 123, 124
Beetles, ocelli in, 125, 126, 159
Bifocal lenses, 153
Binocular vision, 24, 25, 71, 72, 99, 100, 106, 113, 143, 153
Birds, 9, 11, 19, 24, 27, 37, 54, 61, 97–106, 149
  of prey (see also under individual names), 103–105, 152
Bittern, 99, 130
Bleak, 28, 130
Blindness and blind animals, 9, 10
Blind spot, 53, 100

Body colour, changes in, 21, 111
Bowman's membrane, 40
Brachycephalic heads, 71
Brightness, 28
Brow, 20
Bull, vision in, 21, 23, 91
Butterfly, 28, 121, 157
Buzzard, 11

Camel, 64
Camera, 21, 28, 35
Canal of Schlemm, 43, 48, 49
Carnivora, 18
Cartilaginous fishes, 28
Cat, 3, 6, 11, 12, 15–17, 19, 22, 24–26, 48, 58, 64, 75–81
Cataract, 52, 85, 153
Caterpillars, 28, 120
Cave dwellers, 10–12
Central foveae, 53, 54
Chameleon, 22, 116
Children, 2, 24
Choroid, 36, 45–50, 62, 76
Ciliary muscle, 38, 47, 52, 66, 69, 76, 81
  atrophy of, 76, 78
Ciliary processes, 38
Ciliary region, 52
Cod, 153
Colour vision, 1, 2, 27, 64, 69, 91, 93, 96, 107, 114, 115, 117, 123, 130
Compound eyes, 119, 120, 123
  colour perception in, 123
  facets in, 123
Compound lens, 28, 35, 119, 120, 122, 123, 148, 149
Cones (see also Rods and cones), 27, 77, 152
Conjunctiva, 33
Convergence, 20, 21, 24, 105

161

Convexity of cornea, 153
Cormorant, 99, 104
Cornea, 16, 35, 38–42, 52, 61, 82, 83, 95, 107, 124
Corneal shape, 61, 82, 83, 94, 104
Corneal window, 104
Corpora nigra, 84
Cow, 15, 21
Crabs, 8, 135
Crayfish, 135, 136
Crocodile, 116, 117
Crustaceans, 12
Crystalline cone cells (insects), 121
Crystalline lens, 34, 35, 37, 51, 52, 60, 62, 84
Cuttlefish, 139
Cyclops, 8, 9

Dark adaptation, 31, 61–63, 107
Darkness, 4, 5
Decussation of optic nerve, 25, 26
Deep sea fish, 110
Deer, 64, 91
Dependence upon smell and hearing, 52, 142, 149
Dermal receptors, 119
Descemet's membrane, 42
Distance judgement and perception, 21, 78, 123, 152, 155, 156
Diurnal and nocturnal eyes, 28–30, 77, 78
Divergence, angles of, 27, 71, 72, 89, 99, 101, 103
Diving birds, 22, 99, 104, 105, 141, 152
Dog, 1–3, 6, 12, 15, 16, 18–26, 28, 58, 60–65, 70–74, 141–143, 147–149, 151
Dogfish, 130
Dorsal ocelli, 119, 124, 125
function of, 124, 126

Eagles and birds of prey, 151, 152
Earthworms, 135
Eels, 112
Elephant, 15, 16, 21, 92–94, 153
Emmetropia, 67, 68
Environment, 11
Evolution, 8, 11, 13
Eyeball, shape and size, 31, 32, 37, 46, 60, 82, 85, 93, 94, 96, 101, 103
movement of, 21, 23, 46
muscles of, 46

prolapse of, 18, 61
Eyelashes, 32, 37, 61, 85, 86
Eyeless animals, 10
Eyelids, 32, 37, 61, 85
Eyeshine, 29
Eye and camera, 21
Eye moisture, 22
Eye placement, 21–23, 25, 87
Eye position during movement, 92
(see also Parallax)
Eye protrusion (proptosis), 21

Falcon, 140, 152
False gill, in trout, 134
Feelers, 12
Fennec, 65
Fertility and eyesight, 13
Fishes, 13, 27, 37, 83, 107–113, 141, 144–146, 153
Fishes, bony, 110
Flat cornea, 153
Flat fish, 110, 111
eye cycle in, 111
Fleas, 159
Flies, 12, 121, 158
Flying fishes, 112
Flying foxes, 130
Foal, 64
Focal length, 35
Focusing the eyes (see Accommodation)
Foramen of Magenda, 49
Four-eyed fish, 107
Fovea, 53, 54, 62, 102–104
Fox, 64, 142
Arctic, 65
Silver, 64
Foxhound, 142
Fox terrier, 71, 72, 143
Frogs, 19, 28, 105, 117, 118, 141
Frontal vision, 22, 27

Gannet, 22, 105, 152
Gazehounds, 72, 73, 142
Giraffe, 8, 19
Globe of eye, 82
Goose, 17
Greyhound, 3, 68, 70, 156
Goldfish, 146
Guacharo bird, 132
Gulls, 97
Gundogs, 68, 69, 142
Gurnard, 132

Hammer-headed shark, 111
Hare, 21, 26, 81, 134
Hawks, 28, 97, 98, 104, 151, 152
Head shape and vision, 70–72, 87, 88, 90, 92, 94, 99
Hedgehog, 159
Hen, 100, 104
Herring, 132
Hippopotamus, 6, 64, 92, 141, 153
Homing birds, 102, 148
Homing dogs, 147, 148
Horizon, 150
Horse, 15, 16, 20, 21, 26, 64, 65, 80–90
Hounds, 142, 144
Human eye, 1, 2, 6, 15, 22, 24, 25, 31–59, 76, 77, 80
Hyaloid artery, 74, 85
Hyaloid membrane of lens, 47, 52, 73, 74
Hypermetropia, 58, 68, 71, 117
Hypertony, 49
Hypotony, 49

Infra-red rays, 5
Insectivorous animals (birds and mammals), 101
Intracranial pressure, 48–50
equilibrium of, 49
Insects, 12, 119, 126, 149, 157
lateral eyes in, 119, 121
Insect larvae, 126
Iridocytes, 63
Iris, 34, 43, 47–49, 63–66, 84, 107, 121, 124
colour of, 47, 48
Iris propulsion, 118
Jackal, 65
Jumping horses, 82, 87, 91, 155

Kingfisher, 22
Kiwi, 132

Lachrymal gland, 37
Lamina cribrosa, 44
Lamina fusca, 44
Lamprey, 9
Lamps on fishes, 101, 113
Lateral line, on fishes, 107, 111
Lateral ocelli, 119, 121, 126
Layers of retina, 55, 56
Lens capsule, 38, 47, 52
Lens circumference, 52

Lens fibres, 37, 38
Lens growth, 38
Lens nucleus, 37, 38
Lens size, 84
Lens suspension, 62
Lid closure reflex, 32, 33
Light, at depths, 107
Limpet, 137, 141
Lion, 64, 76
Light, absorption of, 4
Light
adaption, 59
admission, 34
definition of, 3
existence of, 4, 5
Light rays, 3–5, 35
infra-red, 5
ultra-violet, 5
under water, 145, 146
Lizards, 28, 54
Tuatera, 9
Lobsters, 135
Long sight, 58

Mackerel, 110
Macula lutea, 12, 54, 62
Meibomian glands, 61, 86
Membrana nictitans, 18, 19, 32, 76, 87, 91, 134
Migrating birds, 148
Mole, 122, 133
Molluscs, 12
Monkeys, 1, 48, 54, 64, 65, 156
Mosquito, 12
Moths, 28
Mouse, 11, 28, 36, 58, 77, 149, 150
Movement perception, 1, 23, 36, 71–74, 123, 149, 151
Mud skipper, 112
Mullet, 110
Mussel, 141
Myopia, 67–68, 71–73

Nautilus, 137
Neck movement, 21, 23, 91
Newt, 117
Night blindness, 30
Night fliers, 104
Nightjar, 103
Norwegian Bream, 108

Objects, distant and moving, 69
Ocelli, 119–126

Octopus, 137
Oil droplets in retina, 28
Ommatidium, 121, 122
Open and closed orbits, 73
Opening eyes, in the young, 73, 74
Opossum, 132
Optic chiasma, 24, 25
Optic disc, 53, 64, 76
Optic divergence, 76
Optic nerve, 25, 52, 104
Ora serrata, 52
Orbit, 15–17, 32, 37
  open or closed, 16–18, 75, 80, 91, 95
Orbital arch, 80
Otter, 135
Owl, 11, 21, 64, 97, 98, 100, 104, 152, 153, 155
Oyster, 137
Ox, 15, 16, 21, 23, 26, 64

Palpebral orifice or fissure, 37, 60, 61, 75
Papilla, 76
Parallactic displacement, 22
Parallax, 22, 157
Paraplasma, 52
Pecten, 100, 102–104
Pectinate ligament, 48
Peripheral vision, 142
Pensioners, 2
Perspective, 78
Pictures, 142
Pig, 15, 16, 26
Pigeon, 99, 102, 103
Pigment cells, 124
Pineal body, 8
Pinhole camera, 78
Plaice and other flat fish, 111, 112
Pollack, 110
Portuguese Man-of-war, 137
Prairie dog, 28
Prawns, 11, 135, 136
Pressure equilibrium, 49
Progressive retinal atrophy, 30, 64, 73, 74
Projectiles, 36
Proptosis, 21
Protractor lentis muscle, in shark, 108
Pupil, 20, 30, 34, 35, 62–64, 76–78, 84, 105
  light changes in, 30, 35, 105
  stenopaic, 66, 105
Puppies, 2, 143

Rabbit, 22, 24, 26, 27, 81, 134
Radar in bats, 21, 130
Ramp retina, 81, 87, 109, 112
Rat, 19, 134
Radiation, 3, 141
Reflection, 4
Refraction, 4
Reptiles, 37, 114–118
Retina, in various animals (see also Ramp retina), 21, 29, 30, 34, 39, 50–56, 62, 63, 67, 69, 72, 74, 76, 87–89, 91, 92, 102–104, 109, 112, 124, 152, 155
Retinal asymmetry, 52
Retinal image, 34, 69, 155
Retinule, 121, 124
Retractor muscle, of eyeball, 32, 105
Rhabdom, 121, 124
Rhinoceros, 92
Rhodopsin, 59
Ringwulst, 98
Robin, 105
Rockfish, 110
Rods and cones, 27, 56–59, 64, 77, 110, 137
Rodents, 133
Ruminants, 91, 92

Salamander, 118
Sclera or sclerotic coat, 44, 45, 51, 83, 105
Sclera ossicle and scleral rings, 83, 94, 104, 105
Seabirds, 102
Seals, 64, 83, 94, 95
Seasonal variations, 84
Second sight, 147
Seeing and perceiving, 9, 34, 35, 69, 70
Seeing stars, 35
Senses and their comparative value (see Smell and hearing)
Shad, 110
Shag, 99, 104, 141, 152
Shark, 108, 110, 133
Sheep, 16, 17, 26, 64, 85
Showjumpers, 82, 87, 91, 155
Shrimps, 11, 135, 136
Sight, 54
Sights or guidelines, 100, 107
Simple eyes, in insects, 124, 126
Skate and rays, 108, 109
Slow worm, 116
Slugs and snails, 11, 137
Smell and hearing, 149, 151, 156, 157

Snakes, 21, 114–118
Snipe, 100, 101
Songbirds, 104
Spaces of Fontana, 42, 48
Sparrow, 96, 105
Spectacles in fishes, 108
Sperm whale, 108
Spectral tarsier, 134
Sphenodon, 9
Spiders, 119–126, 140, 150, 151
hunting, 128
ocelli in, 126
web-weaving, 127
Squid, 110, 137, 138
Squirrel, 74
Stars of Winslow, 76
Starlings, 103, 104
Steering sights, 107
Steopaic aperture, 156
Stereoscopic vision, 25–27, 153
Stickleback, 28
Suspensory ligament of lens, 35, 38, 43, 118
Supersonic vibrations, 21
Suprachoroidal space, 43, 45, 46, 48–50
Supraorbital process, 80
Swallow, 102, 156
Swifts, 102

Tapetum, 28, 29, 36, 76, 92
Tapetum cellulosum, 63
Tapetum nigrum, 64
Tarsier, 7
Tears, 37
Teleosts, 109
Television, 70, 142
Tenon's capsule, 44
Terrapins, 117
Terriers, 142
Third eye, 9
Third eyelid (see also Membrananicti-tans), 18, 19, 32, 76, 87, 91, 104, 105, 134
Tiger, 64, 76
Toads, 117, 118
Tortoise, 117

Touch, sense of, 159
Trout, 124
Tubular eyes, 108
Tunny, 110
Turtle, 19, 28, 105, 117

Ultra-violet rays, 125, 146, 153
Uveal tract, 49

Vibration, 147, 149, 156
Vision, above and below water, 111, 113, 144, 145
day and night, 28, 29
frontal, 71
in the young, 2, 73, 78
monocular and binocular, 36, 71–73, 157
Visual acuity, 11
Visual angle, 24, 69, 95, 97
Visual image, 34
Visual needs, 6–8
Visual purple, 59
Visual violet, 59
Vitamin A, 30, 39
Vitreous body, 47, 52, 124
Vultures, 134

Wading birds, 100, 102
Wingless insects, 121
Wasp, 28, 149
Water voles, 134
Waisted eyes, 98
Wavelength, 5
Whales, 21, 93, 94, 134, 153
Whiskers, 12
White of eye (see Sclera)
Wolf, 64, 67
Woodcock, 100
Worms, 135
eyespots in, 135

Yellow spot (macula lutea), 54

Zonule of Zinn, 37, 66
Zygoma, 18

J5